Everything You've Always
Wanted to Know about

Energy...

but Were Too Weak to Ask

Everything You've Always Wanted to Know about

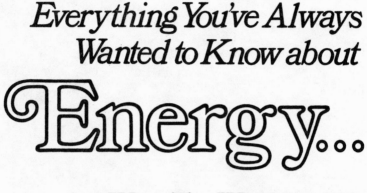

Energy...

but Were Too Weak to Ask

Naura Hayden

HAWTHORN BOOKS, INC.
Publishers/NEW YORK

To Love . . .
Which Is God . . .
Which Is Love

Library of Congress Catalog Card Number: 76-4002
ISBN: 0–8015–8573–2
    5 6 7 8 9 10

WARNING!!!

This book can change your life!

CONTENTS

I Physical Energy

II Mental Energy

III Emotional Energy

FOREWORD

There is not one person on the face of the earth who can't benefit from this book. No matter who you are or what you do—window washer, circus performer, auto mechanic, beautician, dealer (used car or blackjack), debutante, nurse's aide, opera singer, captain (police or tugboat), sanitation worker, veterinarian, ballet dancer, mortician, painter (house or portrait)—this book can change your life; and will, if you apply to your personal life even a small percentage of what you read.

When I finished my last book, I toured all over the United States, appearing on television and radio in most of the big cities and after every show I received an incredible response from the viewers and listeners. The switchboards would be jammed with hundreds of calls, and I would stay after the shows and talk to as many listeners as I could. In fact most of the producers sent me letters attesting that I drew more response than any other guest ever. My great popularity was not due to me, but to my enormous energy. It was unbelievable and a revelation—the one thing most people were interested in was energy. The one thing most people seemed to lack was energy—and they wanted as much info as possible on how to get it.

That was when I decided to write this book, wholly and solely on energy.

I had fortunately found the sources of energy, and I wanted to share them. Now lots of people have said to me, "But I'm sure you've always had energy—you were probably born with it." And I have to reply that that's not true. In fact, just before I first discovered my greatest source of energy, I hit the nadir of energylessness. I was so pooped I could hardly walk across a room. But them days is gone forever.

Read on—and change your life!

Everything You've Always
Wanted to Know about

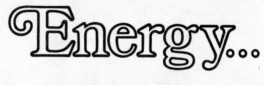

but Were Too Weak to Ask

INTRODUCTION

Are you a victim of the Human Energy Crisis?

Are you drained at the end of the day, and sometimes at the beginning, and do you feel once in a while that life isn't worth living?

Are you tired a lot and do you drink mucho coffee to rev up your motor?

Do you smoke lots of ciggies 'cause they give you the lift you need?

Do you usually have a martini before lunch, and maybe sneak a couple of scotches during the day?

Do you hover between anxiety attacks and bouts of depression that leave you limp as a noodle?

If you answered yes to even one of the above and feel you need to use any kind of "upper" to get you through life, you are definitely a victim of the Human Energy Crisis.

We've heard a lot about energy shortages—gas, oil, coal, electricity, etc.—but the most important energy is the one that runs our personal motors, that gives us a zest for living, that lets us absorb life's problems and keep on going with a smile, knowing that nothing can keep us down.

Look, we all have problems—every one of us. Even the people who look as if they don't, do. A man can have lots of money in the bank, a paid-for mansion and limousine, a terrific job, and his wife—whom he adores—can leave him for a younger stud. It's not the having of problems that can get us, it's how we cope.

And this book will show you how to cope.

It's divided into three sections—physical, mental, and emotional. Once you get your body in shape and then get your mind working right and get your feelings straightened out, you won't believe the amount of energy you'll have to use. We don't realize how tensions (trapped energy) deplete us and make us tired, depressed, and discouraged. I would say at the rate we're going we won't have to worry about gas or oil shortages; we'll be up against a psychiatrist shortage if we don't learn how to conrol our bodies, our minds, and our feelings.

Hundreds of thousands of people are now going to psychiatrists, psychologists, and psychoanalysts to get much-needed help, but the number of needy is growing. There are lots of reasons for this. One is that our diets are so full of junk—candy, booze, coffee, pretzels, etc.—that our bodies are becoming nervous wrecks. Another reason is the rampant moral decay that started in the mid-1950s with the TV quiz scandals and keeps growing all around us, particularly in government. When we see our trusted officials lying, cheating, and believing themselves above the law, it's confusing to us. Why should we be honest when everybody around us isn't? Confusion is one of the most difficult problems to handle and can make a wreck of anyone if we let it.

There's a story told of a little ten-year-old boy back in 1920 who waited outside the courthouse for "Shoeless Joe" Jackson, a player for the Chicago White Sox found guilty of being part of a conspiracy to throw the World Series games in the prior year (and the White Sox were called the Black Sox for some time because of the scandal). Anyway, the little kid walked up to his hero, Jackson, with tears streaming down his face and said, "Say it ain't so, Joe."

That's what we feel like when we're mentally confused about the morality we grew up with. But emotional confusion is even more debilitating. When love gets battered around and our egos get bruised, we can hit the bottom of the barrel. Nothing is tougher to overcome than an emotional clobbering. We feel low and draggy and completely worthless, so we go to a shrink and spend lots of time and money.

It's nice to have someone listen exclusively to our problems for an hour and try to help, but in the long run looking back to mommy and poppy and blaming all kinds of childhood incidents on how awful we feel today isn't really the answer. The reality of the situation is we're emotionally confused today and today is all we have to deal with. Mommy was mean when we were four years old, and poppy beat the hell out of us when we were ten; but we're not four and we're not ten today. We're adults. And when we can emotionally accept the fact that mommy was pretty screwed up herself, and poppy had enormous emotional problems, and they did what they did to us not because we were worthless, but because they were unhappy with themselves and took it out on us, we will have matured enormously. We can still be mad at them and carry around anger for years, but why? It doesn't hurt them, it hurts us.

The only thing we should be concerned with is being able to cope with today. Carrying around anger for things done long ago is illogical and very draining physically, mentally, and particularly emotionally. When you stop and say to yourself—okay, I had lots of unfair things done to me in the past and I'll probably have lots more done in the future; but they're not done deliberately because I'm a bad or inferior person, they're done because lots of the world is confused and neurotic and this makes people selfish— they are really so wrapped up in themselves and their own problems that it's impossible for them to treat others well—you'll be well on the road to overcoming your own Human Energy Crisis.

The whole point of this book is to have you reevaluate habits that drain you of energy—physically, mentally, and emotionally. When your energy level is down, you can't accomplish much and you feel depressed and easily discouraged. But the wonderful thing is that this can be turned around by changing a few bad habits so that an enormous reservoir of energy will be yours to use every moment you need it.

This, then, is a declared war between tension and energy. If one wins, the other has to lose. Read on, and you'll find out how to get rid of tension forever, and how tremendous energy can and will be yours to use to bring you all the things you've always wanted and to give you the happiness you deserve.

I

Physical Energy

1
HOW A MAGIC MILKSHAKE CHANGES TENSION INTO ENERGY

If you were to ask people what they would like if they could have anything in the whole world they wanted, most would say energy. Energy is everything. Energy is great health. Energy, rightly channeled, will get you anything you want—love, friendship, money, power, success, fun—*everything!*

Loaded with energy, you'll feel like a million bucks—you'll feel as though there's nothing you can't do. And you know something? There *will* be nothing you can't do. Anxiety and depression will disappear. Your whole life will change drastically for the better when your body is surging with energy. Believe me, a whole new world of adventure and accomplishment will open up for you.

Now what most people don't know is that energy is not that hard to get once you know the secret.

Before I learned this secret, I smoked a lot and drank cups and cups of coffee to stimulate myself. These were the "uppers" I needed to get through the day. I've since found that most people need these things plus lots of sugar. Sugar is mistakenly thought of as an energy booster; all it does is give you a short spurt up, then you plummet down and get depressed until you eat more sugar—a vicious circle. It's BAD for you—and it's found not only in the sugar bowl, but in cakes, pies, cookies, soft drinks, and in donuts, bread, spaghetti, macaroni and other starchy things.

Before I discovered my great energy secret, I was tired a lot and falling apart physically at a very young age. As I told in my first book, *The Hip, High-Prote, Low-Cal, Easy-Does-It Cookbook*, I'd had canker sores in my mouth dating back to early childhood, and anyone who's had even one knows how painful it is. A canker sore is an ulcer which is in the mouth instead of in the stomach. It's caused by tension—which, in my case, was caused by eating lots of candy, cakes, pies, and sugar in general. Sugar, to be metabolized, must burn up all the B vites in your system in the metabolic process; and let me tell you, a lack of the B vites can leave you very jittery, anxious, and tense, and can cause canker sores, ulcers, heart attacks, acne, and deep psychiatric depressions, among other things.

Hypoglycemia, which is low blood sugar, strangely enough is caused by too much sugar intake in certain individuals. It overstimulates the pancreas to produce too much insulin, which eats up all the sugar in the blood and leaves you with low blood sugar, or hypoglycemia. It's the direct opposite of diabetes, which is too much sugar in the blood caused by the pancreas not secreting enough insulin to keep the blood sugar in balance. Now, unfortunately, hypoglycemia is called "low blood sugar" and of course sounds as if you should eat sugar to correct it. In fact, all the ads saying, "Sugar is energy—kids need it" are very misleading. Sure, sugar's energy—for about ten minutes. Then you plunge down to lethargy and depression.

The true energy food is protein, and the more you eat, the better. If you feel you need energy, take a hard-boiled egg, or a glass of milk, or a handful of sunflower seeds (also FANTASTIC for your eyes!) and see how good you'll feel—and not only for ten minutes, but for hours. You'll have no sharp drop in energy either. It'll be longer lasting and steadier than sugar energy.

I used to eat lots of sugar, drink lots of coffee, and smoke lots of ciggies. I needed these "uppers" to get through the day. These are all drugs 'cause they're habit-forming, but I needed the stimulants, as millions of others do. But I was really lucky. A few years ago I got very sick and had no energy—not even enough to walk across a room—and all the doctors thought I had mono or some such energy-draining disease. They rushed me to the hospital, gave me every test they could think of, and never did

15

find out what the problem was. I hate to repeat myself, but lots of you didn't read my first book, so please excuse my telling again how I got into nutrition.

Anyway, a friend gave me Adelle Davis's book of nutrition, *Let's Eat Right to Keep Fit,* and I recognized so many of my symptoms that I immediately started to take a few vites. Maybe a month or so before I went into the hospital my gums had been bleeding so badly (and had been bleeding on and off since I was a kid) that I went to a periodontist who operated on my gums. Do you believe it! For a very large fee he cut a lot of my gums away. Well, I read in the nutrition book that bleeding gums can be caused by a lack of vitamin C; isn't it a pity my periodontist didn't read this—or maybe if he had he'd be out of business, because if everyone took enough C, maybe he wouldn't have to operate. Anyway, in the hospital my gums started bleeding again and I started experimenting with the C, and miraculously (I thought) the gums stopped bleeding.

Now, everyone has a different body chemistry and different nutritional needs. My requirements for vitamin C are very high, 'cause even though I always drank a glass of orange juice in the morning (100 milligrams of vitamin C), that was never enough for me. I now take 10,000 mgs. every day and my gums are healthy, and all the bruises on my body (another symptom of vitamin C deficiency and embarrassing 'cause all my friends accused me of being a closet masochist) disappeared. I was so astounded by the "cure" I effected when none of the doctors seemed to know what to do, that I began experimenting with other vites.

The book said that powdered torula yeast, or brewer's yeast, is the highest form of all the B vites and a lack of the B vites was causing my canker sores and my tension. So as soon as I got out of the hospital I went right out to a health store and bought the powdered yeast (don't make a mistake and buy baker's yeast—it's bad for you) and started taking it. Well, I can't tell you the energy I began to have. My tension lessened right away; and since tension is trapped energy, all the released energy was mine to use. Everyone who knows me today comments on my enormous energy and great health, and I can honestly say it's not a thing I was born with—I get it from the vites and yeast I take. Some people are born really healthy and stay that way always; they never get sick and need nothing to boost them along. They're fortunate, but there aren't too many of them around. Most of us have to work at feeling great. But let me tell you, it's worth it! I feel so incredibly great every day that nothing—NOTHING—could ever stop me from my "health regime."

When I first started taking the yeast, I put it in orange juice; but the taste bothered me. Not enough to stop me from taking it—as I said, *nothing* could stop me from that—but I used to keep a spoon of peanut butter or a couple of peanuts or a small piece of cheese (only because they have a strong taste) next to me, and I'd quickly pop one of them into my mouth to kill the yeast taste. But then I invented my milkshake, and now I love the taste every morning.

I hereby GUARANTEE that anyone—anyone in the whole

17

world—who takes this every morning for breakfast will start to feel incredibly great and will begin to have enor-mous energy and a terrific sense of well-being. If you tend to be tense and anxious and get depressed easily, you will be amazed at how quickly these problems vanish.

Also you'll start to look better. Your skin and hair will improve. A few months ago I moved into a new apartment and noticed a good-looking young boy of about eighteen or nineteen with the worst case of acne I've ever seen. He was the handyman in the building, and when he came up to fix my refrigerator I started to find out about him (I was born a do-gooder). He was from Bolivia and had come to New York a year before. I told him how handsome he was, or could be, if he cleared up his skin. He said he'd been going to skin specialists for two years—one year in Bolivia and one year in New York. The poor thing didn't earn much as a handyman and was desperately spending what he had to save his skin. The last doctor gave him a special soap, but no results. He had tried antibiotics, salves, creams, etc., etc., etc.

Well, Armando was so desperate, he'd try anything at this point. So I told him about my canker sores and how that's related to acne—both caused by nerves and tension and a lack of the B vites, all making a chemical imbalance in the body. Everyone's symptoms come out in different places. Some of us get heart attacks, others pimples.

I gave Armando a copy of the recipe for my milkshake and he went out on his lunch break and bought all the ingredients. Fortunately he had a blender (he was so desperate he would have bought one if necessary) and began making the milkshake the next morning. You must start out slowly with the powdered yeast; the more deficient you are in the B vites, the slower you must go—if you take too much too soon it'll blow you up like a balloon. So it took three weeks for Armando to get up to four heaping tablespoons of the yeast in his milkshake, but the results were astounding. Almost all the acne had disappeared. There were still a couple of spots on his neck, but his face was clear as a bell. And needless to say, he was really excited. Then about two weeks later I saw him and he had a small recurrence on his face. He told me he had drunk a cola drink the day before, and by night the pimples had come back I told him obviously his body can't handle sugar and to stay completely away from it.

And Armando isn't the only person whose acne cleared up. While in Boston doing a TV appearance ny friend, the late, great writer and wit George Frazier introduced me to the wife of a friend of his. She was in her early forties and had had acne since her teens. I told her what to buy and how to make the milkshake, and a few weeks later she called me in New York to tell me how sensational the milkshake is and how her skin is beautiful for the first time since childhood. Amazing? No, just logical. All we humans are, basically, is a combination of chemicals, and when the chemicals are imbalanced, the skin or hair or eyes or heart go out of commission. Just like a car or any other precision machine.

I happen to be a very logical person. I don't want to

do anything without knowing the reason for it. Everything is cause and effect. It usually takes time between the cause and the effect, and that's generally why we don't pin the effect on the cause or see the reason between the two. But if you put junk into your personal machine, eventually it's gonna conk out. Maybe your eyes will start to go— you'll need stronger glasses; or worse, a cataract operation. Or your teeth will get so many cavities you'll figure you'd rather have them out. Or your skin will get all wrinkly, or pimply. Or your hair will start to thin, or drop out altogether.

Now there is a definite cause and effect between what you put inside your body and what happens on the outside. It's been proven in controlled laboratory experiments (and even if it hadn't, I'm my own proof to myself and you will be to yourself, too) that high amounts of the B vites are vital to good skin, healthy hair, bright eyes, a strong heart, calm nerves, and high energy. So if I tell you my milkshake, which has enormous amounts of the B vites (and it's much better for you than B vitamin pills); plus complete protein (it has 58 grams—the average healthy woman, according to the *U.S. Department of Agriculture Handbook No. 8, Composition of Foods*, needs 60 grams, and the average healthy man needs 70 grams for the *whole day*—and you'll get 58 grams for breakfast *alone*); plus lecithin (extremely important to every cell in your body and the best natural counteracter to cholesterol or fat in your blood); plus calcium in the milk (which every bone in your body needs— young and old alike, but particularly the old, whose bones are usually brittle and porous); plus vegetable oil, which is the principal source of the essential fatty acids, which we need for beautiful skin, glossy hair, healthy glands and hormones, a good sex life, and even for a diet, you can see that you're getting nearly all essential nutrition in a single morning milkshake. Lots of people think they're fat, but they're only waterlogged, and two tablespoons of vegetable oil a day will allow the excess water to leave the body. Always refrigerate vegetable oil once it's opened, and *never* use mineral oil for anything to do with the body —don't swallow it or use it as a body oil. It absorbs vitamins A, D, E, and K, and then washes them out of the body.

I am so positive that anyone, without exception, who drinks this milkshake *every morning* will greatly improve in health and energy within a month of taking it that I offer this written guarantee:

Dear Everybody,

I hereby guarantee that if you drink my milkshake *every day* you will feel enormous improvement in every area of your physical being. You will be more energetic, less anxious and depressed, your skin will improve, you will be better able to cope with any problem, and you will feel better than you've ever felt in your entire life.

You cannot take this without changing your body and your life for the better.

Naura Hayden

I would also like to recommend some vitamins that will work with the milkshake to build fantastic health.

Now here are the recipe and the vites:

First buy powdered torula yeast or brewer's yeast, which has calcium and magnesium added and has a balance of the B vites on the label: vitamins B_1, B_2, and B_6 in the same proportion; that is, 10 mg. B_1, 10 mg. B_2, 10 mg. B_6. There are several brands on the market and they can usually be found in most health food stores. Next buy a jar of granulated lecithin.

Now start the recipe:

NAURA'S DYNAMITE MILKSHAKE

Into a blender pour:

    2 cups skim milk
    1 tablespoon safflower oil
    2 packets (or equivalent) sugar substitute
    1 teaspoon vanilla extract

Start the blender on low and add:

    4 heaping tablespoons powdered yeast
    4 heaping tablespoons lecithin

Stop blender, cover, and put in fridge overnight. (The overnight cold, for some reason, changes the taste of yeast from awful to good.) Next morning put blender on high and whip till foamy for about 30 seconds.

When finished drinking, make tomorrow's batch and put in fridge till next morning.

IMPORTANT

When you start out, use only ½ teaspoon yeast for the first couple of days, then go to 1 teaspoon, then 2 teaspoons, then 1 tablespoon, then 1 heaping tablespoon, etc., till you reach 4 heaping tablespoons (about 3 weeks).

You should start right out with 4 heaping tablespoons of lecithin.

VITAMINS TO TAKE

Buy:
Vitamin A—10,000 units
Vitamin C—500 mgs. ascorbic acid
Vitamin D—2,500 units natural
Vitamin E—400 units mixed tocopherols
Dolomite (calcium & magnesium)—calcium 130 mg.
magnesium 78 mg.

Every morning (with yeast milkshake) take:
    2 Vitamin A
    4 Vitamin C
    1 Vitamin D
    1 Vitamin E
    10 Dolomite

Every evening (after dinner) take:
   2 Vitamin A
   4 Vitamin C
   1 Vitamin D
   1 Vitamin E
   10 Dolomite

Every body is individual. You can increase the vitamin C (if you still catch a cold or virus) and the vitamin E (which works as an oxygenizer—good for the heart and other muscles). You get an enormous amount of the B vitamins in the yeast. Do not increase the amount of vitamins A or D.

Powdered yeast is all protein, no fat. Don't take uncooked baker's yeast by mistake. Powdered yeast has more B vitamins and more all-around nourishment than any other food. Two heaping tablespoonfuls have 20 grams of perfect, complete protein, which is as much as an average serving of beef. Yeast is probably the best-known food for beautifying the skin, and I don't know a man or woman, young or old, who wouldn't give a lot for great skin. Yeast is a fabulous way to diet. Take it just before a meal and you won't overeat—you'll push the food away 'cause you'll be stuffed!

Lots of people ask me if the milkshake is fattening. No, it isn't. First of all, it's a meal in itself, so don't eat other things with it. Just consider it your total breakfast (or lunch), and you won't gain weight; but you will gain mucho energy. I'm a slender person, but I'm prone to put on weight, so I really watch not only the quality of the food I put in my mouth but also the quantity.

The reason for starting out slowly with the yeast is that usually a person deficient in the B vites—as almost everybody is—has incomplete digestion; but in a few days you'll have absorbed enough Bs from the yeast so you can slowly take more and more. And remember, the more you need the yeast (B vites) the more reaction you might have at the beginning. In other words, an extremely nervous person might have to stay a week on half a teaspoon of yeast before graduating to a teaspoon. If you do have a reaction (like not digesting it fully) and you blow up, recognize this as a good sign. You are desperately in need of it, so for heaven's sakes don't stop—just slow down the amount of yeast.

If for some reason you don't think you can tolerate milk, use any juice instead; but you lessen the complete protein by 18 grams, and of course you get less calcium too. It just isn't as effective without milk, so if you can, learn to love milk and use it in the shake.

This must be taken every day without exception. If you have to go out of town overnight, take it in a thermos. If you go away for a longer period of time, pack your blender, yeast, vanilla, and lecithin. Any hotel or motel can give you the milk, oil, and sugar substitute. I've traveled over Europe, across the United States, and even down to Buenos Aires and Rio with all my supplies in my bag. It's like taking an electric shaver or an iron—if it's a necessity, you'll pack it. And you'll start to feel so great, you'll treat yeast like a necessity—'cause it is!

I learned about lecithin from Linda Clark's terrific book, *Stay Young Longer*. She relates how lecithin has been found to reduce cholesterol and help dissolve plaques already in the arteries; to lower blood pressure in some people; to produce more alertness in older people; to increase the gamma globulin in the blood, which fights infection; to help acne, eczema, and psoriasis; to soften aging skin and keep the skin in good shape while reducing; to be a tranquilizer and help nervous exhaustion; to act as a brain food and help rebuild brain cells (and one study showed that the brain of an insane person had only half as much lecithin in it as a normal brain); to be a sexual aid and restore sexual powers (seminal fluid contains much lecithin); to aid glandular exhaustion and nervous and mental disorders, to redistribute weight, shifting it from unwanted parts to parts where it's needed; to help in the assimilation of vitamins A and E; to prevent and cure fatty liver; to lengthen the lives of animals and to produce healthier coats and more alertness; and to lower the requirement of insulin in diabetics (with the additional help of vitamin E).

Now let me explain about the vitamins so you'll know why you're taking them and what they'll each do for you.

Vitamin A is essential to good skin—it prevents and clears up skin infections; it makes shiny hair; it improves day vision and particularly night vision; it promotes cell growth; and it aids in resisting infections. Vitamin A and vitamin E work together, because without vitamin E vitamin A is destroyed by oxygen. Vitamin A is found in green and yellow vegetables and apricots. The National Research Council recommends 5,000 units of vitamin A a day, but I take 50,000 units a day and believe that 25,000 units a day should be a minimum. Vitamins A and D are the only vitamins that can be toxic, but only in massive doses. According to E. Lehman and H. G. Rapaport in the *Journal of the American Medical Association* 94 (1940), children have been given 300,000 units of vitamin A daily over long periods without apparent harm, and physicians have recommended curative doses of 200,000 units daily for months. And according to F. Bicknell and F. Prescott in *The Vitamins in Medicine*, vitamin A toxicity can be prevented or corrected by an increased vitamin C intake.

I've done television shows with a few doctors who scare people into thinking that anything over 5,000 units of vitamin A can be harmful, but they've all been amazed when I've pointed out that a seven-ounce portion of beef liver gives you 106,800 units of vitamin A, according to the *United States Department of Agriculture Handbook No. 8, Composition of Foods*, put out by the Agricultural Research Service of the United States; and a 3½-ounce serving of spinach or other cooked greens give 12,000 units of vitamin A. One serving of yams, sweet potatoes, yellow squash, carrots, broccoli, string beans, or apricots supplies 5,000 units of vitamin A. So obviously 5,000 units is not the limit. Many people who know nutrition try to eat liver a few times a week, and I know some people who eat it every day for lunch or dinner; it's the most nutritious meat you can eat. As I said, I take 50,000 units of vitamin A a day, and have for years, and I'm bursting with health and energy.

The B vitamins are B_1, B_2, B_6, B_{12}, biotin, folic acid, inositol, niacin, pantothenic acid, and PABA (para amino benzoic acid). Science is finding there are other B vitamins, and has recently isolated two, B_{15} (pangamic acid) and B_{17}. All the B vitamins are water-soluble and can't be stored in the body, so they should be taken every day. They are synergistic, which means that one alone or several together increase the need for the rest of them. They are necessary for steady nerves, healthy eyes, and skin—and the richest source of all the B vites is powdered yeast.

Vitamin C is ascorbic acid, and Nobel Prize winner Linus Pauling recommends 3,000 mgs. a day; but I take 10,000 mgs. a day and have for years. If I feel a cold coming on, I up my dosage to as high as 80,000 mgs. a day, and I haven't had one day of sickness since I started this. Before I discovered vitamin C, I had colds and viruses at least eight or ten times a year which bedded me each time for at least three days, and sometimes as long as a week. Now every person has different nutritional requirements, and mine obviously are very high. If you never get a cold, you probably need much less than I; but vitamin C is water-soluble and can't be stored in the body, so any excess is flushed out, and the body tissues should be saturated with it every day. I figure better you waste a little and make sure your cells are saturated than make a mistake in the other direction and not have enough. Be sure you drink lots of liquids when you take large amounts of vitamin C.

One glass of orange juice supplies 100 mgs. of vitamin C, and the only way to get much more is with ascorbic acid tablets, which are much less expensive than the "natural" vitamin C tablets; and according to Linus Pauling there is no difference chemically. When a virus or foreign substance tries to invade the body, it attacks the vitamin C, destroys it, and is destroyed by it in the process (the reason for massive daily doses). It works best when calcium is present in the body, so be sure to drink lots of milk or take calcium/magnesium tablets every day. Smoking uses up 25 mg. of vitamin C per cigarette, so if you smoke or use aspirin or antihistamine, or any drug remedy, or have any allergy, take plenty of vitamin C to detoxify them all.

There's a marvelous book out written by Irwin Stone, the biochemist who started Linus Pauling on vitamin C, and to whom Pauling dedicated his book *Vitamin C and the Common Cold*. The name of Irwin Stone's book is *The Healing Factor: "Vitamin C" Against Disease*, and in it he explains that vitamin C isn't really a vitamin at all, and that every animal on earth except man, the monkey family, a fruit-eating bat in India, and the guinea pig manufacture ascorbic acid in their liver. Through some mutation millions of years ago we lost this ability, and we die within weeks if we don't add some ascorbic acid to our diet. Irwin Stone recommends that a baby of one year receive 1 gram (1,000 mg.) of vitamin C daily, a child of four, 4 grams, a child of ten, 10 grams—and then you should stay on 10 grams a day for the rest of your life.

Science has proved that many signs thought to be standard for old age are merely disease symptoms. Children of eight or ten with scurvy (vitamin C deficiency) lose their teeth and have humped-over shoulders and saggy, wrinkly skin. Take a look at photos of scurvied kids and you'll see what I mean. They honestly look like old midgets —it's incredible. One of the first signs of scurvy is bleeding gums; bruises on the body are another sign. So if you bruise easily or your gums ever bleed, up your intake of vitamin C until both symptoms disappear.

Vitamin D is known as the sunshine vitamin and helps the body absorb calcium and retain it; without vitamin D, much calcium is lost. Foods contain little, so many people are terribly deficient and don't know why they are so nervous. Vitamin D can't be absorbed without fat or oil, so take it after a meal that includes some oil —like your milkshake! Vitamin D, like vitamin A, can be toxic, but only in massive doses. I take one 50,000-unit capsule of vitamin D a week with my milkshake, usually on Saturday or Sunday. I get it through a pharmacist friend of mine. Dr. J. A. Johnston of the Henry Ford Hospital in Detroit researched vitamin D, and his studies indicate that an adult can profit by taking at least 4,000 units daily. I take over 7,000 units a day (50,000 a week), and since this amount is not toxic I think most people should do the same.

Vitamin E is an oxygenizer, and it helps all the muscles in the body by lowering the demands of oxygen. With increased oxygen, the heart doesn't have to work as hard. Vitamin E is also known as the sex vitamin and helps produce normal sex hormones. Vitamin E adds oxygen to the brain and has been used to help mentally retarded children. Dr. Del Giudice, chief of child psychology, National Institute of Public Health, Buenos Aires, Argentina, has given mentally retarded children 2,000 to 3,000 units of vitamin E daily for many years with surprisingly successful results and no evidence of toxicity.

Wheat germ, wheat-germ oil, and soybean oil are the richest sources of vitamin E. I take 3,200 units a day, but I suggest you start out with 800 units; or, if you want to start out very slowly, 400 units.

Dolomite is a mixture of calcium and magnesium, so I'll explain both. If you want calm nerves, calcium is for you. Most of the calcium in the body is in the teeth and bones, but the rest is used by the nervous system. For calcium to be absorbed in the body, you must take some fat or oil with it; use whole milk instead of skim, or if you drink skim milk, have a salad with oil in the dressing, or something else with oil in it. Magnesium is a mineral also important to the nervous system. It's found in green leaves, but it's lost in discarded cooking water. I take a lot of dolomite—ten pills after each meal, and ten with some plain yogurt before I go to bed. If I ever wake up in the middle of the night and can't get back to sleep, I go to the kitchen and take ten more dolomite with plain yogurt—yogurt is predigested milk and works quicker than plain milk. In minutes I'm zonked—so relaxed you can't believe it. Try it if you have a sleeping problem.

The first time I did Regis Philbin's TV show in Los Angeles, he kept asking me about all my energy and I told him about my milkshake. He asked me to send him the recipe, which I did. The next time I did his show he told me how sensational he felt 'cause he'd been taking it every day. Red Buttons changed his life through vitamins and terrific nutrition. If you ever meet him ask him about it. He can talk for an hour on it. Just notice how young he looks, and you'll know it works.

I used to see Ali MacGraw a lot in a West 57th Street health store in New York. She's really hip to health foods, which give her enormous energy and keep her so sensationally healthy looking.

Sheila MacRae is gorgeous, ageless, and a grandmother. Frank Sinatra calls her the oldest innocent in the world; and he may be right, because she's adorable, and she really concentrates on her nutrition. She takes 5,000 mg. of vitamin C every day, plus yeast, lecithin, kelp, dolomite, vitamins A and D, protein tablets, and lots of yogurt. Her body's in terrific shape, she's energetic and has a great personality, and she attributes a lot of her success to taking care of herself nutritionally.

To me, great beauty is health. I'd rather see a man or woman with less than perfect features but with great skin and color, shiny hair, sparkling eyes, and a zest for life than a man or woman with perfect features but none of the above. How can you be gorgeous if you feel draggy? It ain't easy. But it is easy to change your diet pattern. Actually what I'm talking about isn't a diet—it's a way of life. If you start looking at yourself objectively, you realize that everything you put in your tummy is a cause and will have an effect—some immediate, like headaches, pimples, canker sores, and some long-range, like ulcers, a stroke, a heart attack, or any disease that strikes an older body—and we all get there eventually. After years of mistreating your beautiful body, can you blame it for falling apart? But the beauty part is that it's never too late. Don't hide from your body, 'cause it sure can't hide from you. Even if you've been mistreating yourself for years and years, stop—NOW—and start a new way of life— one that I *guarantee* will make you happier, healthier, and lots more energetic!

2
STOP PEOPLE POLLUTION!

You can have four wives, two husbands, twelve kids, a thousand pals—but you have only one body, and that's gotta last a lifetime. So why do we feel so guilty about taking care of it? It's one thing to stare passively in a mirror for four hours and another to be sure to put only health-building things into the machine. Because it is a machine. Not the mind or the soul—but the body is a machine, and it needs good fuel.

Do you know what would happen if you put sand in your car's gas tank? Or water? Or if you let it sit for months without moving it? It wouldn't run. And the same thing happens with your body. Put booze and pretzels and candy bars in your stomach and smoke in your lungs, and you're gonna slow down and eventually stop much sooner than you would if you kept that junk out. Or if you don't walk or do any exercise or play any physical games, your muscles will shorten or shrivel up. Is it too much to like yourself? To like your body? To like it so much that you really care for it the way you'd care for a Rolls-Royce? Or a Secretariat? Or a Steinway piano? There are lots of ways to take good care of the body, to treat it like a costly machine, and to look at it objectively, unemotionally as the complex machinery that it is.

There's a terrific yoga breathing exercise that's so simple it takes only about five minutes to do, but it clears out all the stale air and fills the lungs with good ol' oxygen and makes you feel sensational. There are slantboards and a few very easy morning exercises for people who get bored doing exercise (like me!)—these take less than five minutes. Lots of former sports stars, like Frank Gifford and Don Maynard, still take good care of their bodies, so why not you? And the terrific thing is, if you do start taking care of your body, you'll not only feel great, you'll start to look a lot better too, and nobody's going to fight *that.*

The very first thing you do in bed in the morning as soon as you wake up is slowly exhale through your mouth all the stale air from your lungs, and when you reach the point where there's not a drop of air left, hold it for five seconds, then very slowly inhale through your nose until your lungs are completely full, then hold for a count of fifty and repeat this four times. By the end of the fifth exhale, your mind will be so alert you'll be startled. What a terrific way to start the day.

Now, exercise can be pretty boring. All my life I hated the thought of it, so naturally I never did it. Of course, with all my newfound energy I did lots of nonexercise activities like walking a lot to appointments, running a lot to late appointments, playing tennis, etc., but until I got a slantboard I never did plain old exercises. And I still don't really, but I've found a few very short and sweet things to do to start the day, and since I've started them, I never miss 'em. And they're for specific things—like twenty sit-ups on el slanto to guarantee a flat tummy for-ever—it takes a fast two minutes, and it's like doing one hundred on the flat, unslanted floor.

Then I stay on the board another two minutes while the blood and oxygen go to my brain, and I quietly get myself together for the day. I think about my source, which is love, which is God, and I visualize my family and all my friends and wish only love and joyous things for them, and then I think about a few people who aren't too loving toward me or who have tried to hurt me, and I wish them love too. When you can do this you realize no one can really ever hurt you. It's only your reaction to a person or a thing that can hurt you. So if you can relax a few moments and think positively about everyone you've ever met, and imagine that you're holding the world in your two hands and wishing it love and everyone on it love and success—what a feeling of power! It may seem silly, but as an actress, my imagination is so sharp that this is easy for me to do, and it will be for you, too, given a little practice.

It works for me. Like with the man at the watch manufacturing place who was Charlie Charming on the phone, but when I went over to pick up my watch and found he was charging me for something that was defective in it and I refused to pay, he became really nasty, and I left his place watchless and upset. Now, I don't like to ever be upset 'cause it keeps my body from being relaxed and causes tension and it never hurts the other person—it only hurts me. So I came home, lay down on my slantboard and imagined the man's face and wished him love. I told myself that he was only doing his job. He felt he was right, and fear or tension or a fight with his wife kept him from being more charming with me in person. After this, even though the thought of seeing him again wasn't thrilling to me, I was very relaxed about him and he couldn't upset me again.

And he didn't. When I returned I gave him my biggest smile, and he actually smiled back, and we worked out the watch problem. Maybe he had time to figure out he shouldn't make enemies out of his customers or maybe my love waves reached him—I don't know. But I do know that I stayed relaxed, so even if he had stayed nasty, it wouldn't have bounced back off me—it would have been absorbed in my relaxed attitude.

If you do this with anyone who is rude to you, or people who raise their voices or yell at you, or even those who refuse to speak to you, your whole reaction to them will change. And life seems to be more reacting than acting. The reason I put love in this chapter is that while you're purging your lungs of stale air, you're purging your mind of negativism, and you can't really change your life until you become positive and release all your negative emotions.

Another terrific thing to do in the morning before work is to run, or jog, in place. I was given a very in-expensive jogging device made of foam rubber and springs, measuring about two feet by three feet, and every morning I jog on it. I started with 100 jogs and have worked up to 250 so far (250 jogs on it is like 500 on the floor because the foam rubber and springs make it seem you're running uphill). I'm panting so heavily when I'm finished (it takes about three minutes) that I walk around my apartment and it seems as if my breath is coming from my toes—it feels sensational!

These few exercises give you so much extra oxygen you gotta feel good, and of course, once you start taking the milkshake you'll have so much extra energy you won't be able to sit still.

I decided to ask a few super-energetic people who accomplish lots of good things what they do for exercise. Virginia Graham is one of the most alive people in the whole world, and one of the best television interviewers in the medium. I know—I was on her television show

"Girl Talk" six times. To know her is to love her. She walks miles every day. Of course New York is a great place to walk—there's so much to see and do on every block. But wherever you live, once you get the energy you'll start to walk. And Virginia does most of her own housework 'cause she figures it's forced exercise with all the bending and pushing, etc.

David Susskind is loaded with energy. He takes yeast and vites and always had lots of energy in the daytime for his work, but he used to fold up after dinner. Then he cut out most carbohydrates (desserts, sugar, bread, etc.) and upped his protein intake. Now he's rarin' to go day or night. For exercise, in the morning he runs in place for ten minutes, does push-ups and knee bends, and two or three times a week he goes to a gym during his lunch or after work, does forty minutes of gymnastics, and swims for twenty minutes.

Serge Obolensky, a Russian nobleman transplanted to America many years ago, is an amazing man. He's always been in the center of New York's social life, and now, at a very advanced age, he's incredibly young. He's never let his weight get out of hand, and his posture is incredible. He does ten minutes of yoga every day, which he started in the 1940s when he met a woman teacher of yoga; at first he thought it was silly, but he tried it once and felt so much better that he's been yoga-ing ever since.

One day at lunch at the Lambs Club I was asked to be the mascot for a celebrity baseball team, and I said absolutely not—I would play ball or nothing. They accepted me at my word that I can play, and I became second baseperson for the first inning and relief pitcher when Jim Bouton had to leave to go back to CBS. As pitcher I won the game 15–12 over the mayors of New Jersey (who played for blood, let me tell you—it was televised, and I think they visualized every voter watching them). Jim had a newfound respect for me and woman-kind when he found out later I'd won the game; and I was the only woman on the team. I asked him if he still played ball or did other exercises, and he said he does isometrics every morning when brushing his teeth and shaving, he walks a lot around the studio, and he is very active at home so he burns up lots of energy. His body is in great shape, so he's doing something right.

Walter Cronkite loves to dance, which is a sensational way to exercise to music. Walter happens to be a Charles-ton champion and will whip into a frenzied solo at any opportunity—and he's great! Walter also plays tennis twice a week in the wintertime and every single day in the summer. He looks younger in person than on TV—he's got terrific coloring from being so physically active.

Arlene Dahl exercises every day—she stretches and bends and plays many sports as often as she can. She swims, skis, plays tennis, snorkles, and next she's going to learn riding. Every year she learns one new sport.

Frank Gifford does seventy-five push-ups every day and then does isometrics for the rest of his body.

Johnny Carson lifts weights every day.

Mitzi Gaynor jogs before breakfast every day—she

either runs through her house, up and down stairs, or she runs in place, and she's been doing it for the last fifteen years. Sometimes she runs with a girl friend through Beverly Hills—and she's one of the few entertainers who can sing a song after doing a wild dance number. Generally dancers are so pooped it takes minutes before they can talk easily, much less sing.

Hildegarde, the incomparable chanteuse, has been around for sixty-eight years, and I still find that hard to believe. She has the skin of a woman twenty-five years younger, and a glorious figure—but she really works at it. Every day, without exception, she does ten minutes worth of stretching and bending to keep her body in shape. She also does facial isometrics, which keep her facial muscles firm. If everyone would eat wisely and exercise every day, and look at Hildegarde, as an example, the fear of old age would disappear, 'cause she ain't old—she really looks young.

And look at Doris Day—in her fifties and she truly looks in her early thirties. I've spotted her many times tooling around Beverly Hills on her bicycle. So you don't *have* to look like a prune as you get older.

One of the worst things a person can do is smoke, particularly cigarettes, 'cause they're always inhaled (cigars and pipes are worse for the people *around* the smoker). Dr. J. J. Burrascano, a New York chest physician, says that the rate of increase of lung cancer in the past forty years has been tremendous, fifteen times, and that it is clear that it is largely the result of personal pollution, namely smoking.

Smoking is the one thing most responsible for aging, and it definitely causes wrinkles of the skin and destroys nerve tissue. Dr. H. Daniell tested more than 1,000 people and found there's a definite cause and effect between smoking and the formation of wrinkles.

Lots of people feel that it's too late to stop smoking —that all the damage is already done. But this is wrong. Dr. Oscar Auerbach, M.D., reports, "We have additional evidence that when you stop painting the tracheobronchial tree with a carcinogenic agent, those cells that are progressing toward cancer shrivel away, contract, disintegrate, and disappear."

Three large groups of people were tested in a recent study—nonsmokers, heavy smokers, and heavy smokers who had quit cigarette smoking at least six months ago. There was no difference between nonsmokers and heavy smokers who had quit.

If I can quit, anyone can. I used to smoke at least one pack a day—yech! But I must admit I don't think I could have stopped without the yeast milkshake to calm my nerves. It really helped incredibly. Because ciggies are an addiction—no less than heroin or any other drug. It's just that you can function with ciggies, and you can't with heroin. But the damage to your body cells is enormous. You will go through actual withdrawal—ask anyone who's kicked the habit—but the yeast will help pull you and your nerves through.

Cigarettes put an incredible stress on your body. And with all the stresses of life—air pollution, the struggle for self-preservation, trying to earn a living, the need for self-expression, the emotional problems in love affairs, the bust-ups of families—why add one of the biggest stresses of all? And one of the most aging.

Hans Selye, professor of medicine at the University of Montreal, is the widely accepted authority on stress, and according to the many autopsies he's performed, he's never seen a person die of old age. He says we die because one vital part has worn out too early in proportion to the rest of the body. The biologic chain that holds our cells together is only as strong as its weakest vital link. When one of the vital links breaks, our parts can't be held together as a living body. And if we smoke, we not only gravely damage the lungs and heart, we damage every cell in our body.

Getting back to exercise, Dr. Joyce Brothers swims for one hour every evening. She lives in New York in an apartment house that has a pool in the basement, and she really takes advantage of it. She also plays tennis and golf as often as she's able. I guested with Sergio Franchi on Joyce's television show, and she's not only a brilliant woman, but she surprised everyone with her charm and personality. She takes very good care of herself, never puts junk in her body, and is a lot of fun to be around.

Howard Cosell is a dynamo—he's on the go all the

time. He walks to most of his appointments around New York City, and he says this is more exercise than most exercisers do.

Buddy Rich practices karate every day by himself. He's so good at it that he's a black belt, the ultimate in karate. He also plays golf and races sports cars. I don't think they're too physically strenuous, but I guess the karate makes up for it.

So to keep our beautiful machines in great working order, we know we must keep the junk foods out, sugar out, smoking out, and put in only energy-building foods, which will give us such incredible energy that we won't be able to sit and wait for things to happen—we'll feel like walking, playing sports, exercising, and just *doing!* All of this will fill our lungs with good old oxygen (try to exercise or play either indoors or in unpolluted areas), and will make us really glad we're alive.

Here's a list of exercises you can try at home:

1. Running in place
2. Jogging from room to room
3. Sit-ups on a slantboard
4. Dancing by yourself to rock music (make sure the blinds are down!)
5. Knee bends
6. Stretching all muscles
7. Skipping rope
8. Chinning on a chinning bar (You can buy an inexpensive portable bar that twists and untwists in a doorway—and women can begin work on the bar

by just hanging by their arms and gradually trying
to raise themselves up. A great-looking girl friend
of mine is actually able to chin herself, but it took
months of daily practice—and she wound up with
a more fabulous bustline than she started with. I'm
only at the point of jumping up and chinning myself
—I can't start from scratch and raise myself yet. I
have the bar in my kitchen doorway, and it's great
at a party. *Everyone* tries to see if he or she can
chin better than everyone else, and it's really fun!)

Start slowly on any of these exercises. The first day
use maybe thirty seconds or a minute, and gradually
work up to a few minutes.

Now of course if you have a swimming pool nearby,
that's the greatest exercise—swimming uses every muscle,
and it's fun. And tennis is great; it's my favorite. After an
hour of batting balls around I feel so fantastic I could start
all over for the second hour. Volleyball in the summer,
ice skating in the winter—there's always something to play
at besides bridge or gin rummy.

Another fun thing to do is join a dance class. There's
modern dance or ballet—it's inexpensive, and sometimes
things done with a group are more exciting than done
alone. If you know anyone who dances in a class, ask if
he or she doesn't feel terrific after an hour of dancing.
Even if you're beat and exhausted when you walk into
class, you'll feel energized and much better after the work-
out than you did before. The only proof will be when you
try it, but asking around will help you realize it's true.

When you've got as much energy as you will have when you start to down the yeast, lecithin, and vites, your body will begin to feel so powerful and sensational that you'll wonder how you ever existed before you learned how to really *live*.

3
SEX:
IT ISN'T
EVERYTHING,
BUT WHAT ELSE
COMES AS CLOSE?

What's the big fuss all about anyway! Sex is only an expression of love. God knows we need more love in the world—and what a super way to express it, to show that we care for one another. There's a terrific bumper sticker out now—"Remember when the air was clean and sex was dirty?" Well, sex was *never* dirty. A few misguided souls might have *thought* it was bad and evil, but they wouldn't even have been here if their mommies and daddies hadn't fornicated, so what do *they* know?

Isn't it a pity that something so terrific should make some people feel so guilty? But some people feel guilty about waking up in the morning—and if they'd only realize that sex is not only fun, but slimming! Sex regulates your heartbeat, breathing, glands, muscles—*everything*—and you'll never feel closer to a person, in fact physically you can't *get* closer, than while making love. If God is love, and all religions preach this, and sex is an expression of love (what else could it be—an expression of hate?) then an expression of God is sex—or making love.

Now, everybody's got the same basic equipment. Every man has more or less the same genitals. Some are longer and fatter, some are shorter and thinner, but basically the same shape. All women have breasts and vaginas—some firmer, some smaller, but basically the same shape. So what's the fuss? It's what's upstairs in the head that's important; that's what turns us on. Without a healthy sex life, a person can't be truly healthy.

If, when you disrobe in front of your love, you have a body that's bursting with health and energy, a body with no extra fat, only what makes for nice curves, a body that says, "Touch me—I want to be loved," a body that you're proud of, you're going to want to take care of that body sexually; and making love is one of the most important ways of keeping in shape physically.

Our physical, mental, and emotional selves are all tied together, and when you make sure to feed and exercise and love your body with only the best, your body will be beautiful and make you happy. As long as you care for it, it will help keep you mentally and emotionally happy too!

A while ago I was involved with a gorgeous male—he

looked like a Greek god. His body and face were nearly perfect; but what a bore. His mind was slow, and he was very involved with himself. Not too long after I stopped seeing him, I met one of the physically ugliest men I've ever seen. His nose was huge, and the rest of his features were all uneven—but *que hombre!* He was sharp and funny and kind and all those terrific qualities that endear one person to another. The only reason I tell of these two guys is because the first had great equipment but didn't know or care how to use it and was a total bore; and the second's equipment seemed totally unexciting, but he sure turned me on (*mucho macho*, as the Norwegians say).

So sex, and all the excitement that goes with it, is primarily mental. If someone turns us on mentally, the face and body are secondary.

Isn't it sad that something so beautiful is so misunderstood. Some people seem able to tolerate violence in movies—killings, bloody murders, knife fights, war monstrosities—but get all shook up over a nude male or female body, and God forbid they should make love on the screen. Now this is only my opinion, but I can't understand parents not worrying over their kids seeing hatred and men killing other men and decapitating bodies, yet getting upset over sex on screen. Sex is an outcome of love—even animal sex has behind it the subconscious desire to procreate—whereas murder and violence is the outcome of only hate and fear.

Repressed sex is tension, and tension is the enemy of energy.

Dr. Frank Slaughter says in *Medicine for Moderns:*

It is far more important that the sex impulse be recognized and treated fairly than any question of morality. A person who satisfies his sex impulse in what society likes to call immorality, and has no further trouble with it, is far better off than the moral person who becomes obsessed with ideas of cleanliness and godliness, in compensation for sex urges which he or she refuses to recognize, resulting in invalidism, and even insanity. Too much morality is probably worse, psychologically, than too much immorality.

I have my own philosophy on why we've been so repressed sexually. I believe millions of years ago we ate berries and nuts and vegetation, as monkeys do today. One day one of us killed an innocent animal and ate it. The guilt had to go somewhere for something we subconsciously knew to be wrong, so it went to the most pleasurable undertaking—sex. That's when the "Eve and the serpent" nonsense came in. I believe that the sin was killing, but as I said, this is only my opinion (the word "sin" comes from the Latin *sine*, which means "without" —without God, or love).

There was a story not too long ago in *Time* magazine about an aboriginal tribe found in the rain forest in the Philippines. Time had stood still for this tribe. They were exactly the same as they had been for perhaps thousands of years. They had never been seen by an outsider; and they, of course, knew nothing about civilization in the outside world.

They are called the Tasaday, and those who have observed them and worked with them call them the gentle Tasaday. They eat no meat and they live on fruits, nuts, vegetables, roots, and berries. The most amazing thing about them is that they show no negative emotions. They are very happy people. They are never angry or fearful or jealous, and they are very philosophical and poetic. They are also very loving toward each other. It may or may not be later proved, but I do believe this lack of negativism is because they don't kill animals and they don't eat meat. As I said before, this is only my opinion, but there are many other people who share this opinion.

There is nothing on earth that feels as good physically —that gives as much joy—as making love (or having sex) with a loved one. And when one is guilt-ridden, we lay it on the greatest pleasure. After all, if I'm guilty, I'm not worthy of pleasure.

Now if eating meat were necessary for our well-being, that would be one thing. But it's not. I haven't eaten one piece of any meat for over eight years, and I'm the healthiest person I know. I'm living proof that you don't need meat to be energetic or healthy. I eat lots of eggs (they're loaded with lecithin which counteracts and emulsifies any cholesterol, and they're the best complete protein you can eat—read chapter 2, "Egg-o-mania," in *The Hip, High-Prote, Low-Cal, Easy-Does-It Cookbook*), cheese, cottage cheese, nuts, sunflower seeds (delish mixed with cottage cheese and sugar substitute—tastes better 'n' ice cream and *loaded* with complete prote). I also drink a quart of milk a day—two cups in my milkshake and yogurt or milk again later in the day.

This isn't to say that meat isn't complete protein. It is, and I'm not trying to get anyone to stop eating it. I do my thing and you do yours. I've never ever suggested that anyone stop eating meat. But if you have considered it, I just want you to know you can be very healthy without it, as I am.

Dr. Benjamin S. Frank is the pioneer in nucleic acid and nucleic acid therapy on aging. I just recently found out from him that powdered yeast is not only the highest form of the B vites (the reason I started taking it), but also the highest and best form of nucleic acid in the diet. Now nucleic acid is the blueprint in every cell. It contains DNA and RNA, and as the cell gets older the nucleic acid gets weaker, and the blueprint makes the next cell a little less young. But when you take in foods high in nucleic acid, the blueprint will stay stronger and each new cell will be more like the one that expired and will be younger and more energy-filled. Besides yeast, seafood is extremely high in nucleic acid, while meat has practically none. Meat is complete protein, but so are seafood, milk, eggs, cheese, yeast, etc., so if you want to keep your cells young and energetic, eat less meat and more seafood and other complete proteins. I stopped eating meat only because I love animals, but I honestly think I'm healthier because of it.

And of course the more energy your cells contain, the more energetic and healthy you'll be. And the more energetic and healthy you are, the sexier you'll be. A great sex drive is a sign of great health. I've never known a successful person, male or female, who didn't have enormous drive, and that drive to success is also a sex drive channeled in a different direction.

Dr. Arnold A. Hutschnecker, internationally known psychotherapist and writer (*The Will To Live*, now in its twenty-fifth successful year, *Love and Hate In Human Nature*, *The Will To Happiness*, and his latest, *The Drive For Power*) is well known for his editorials in the *New York Times* dealing with psycho-political issues and the role psychiatry should have in choosing political leaders. He coined a new term for study called "psychopolitics." Dr. Hutschnecker, who has also written many other articles on depression, tension, and anxiety in leading magazines and other publications, believes that the repression of sex, which is a most basic human need, causes many neurotic problems, and that sexual satisfaction secures a state of well-being and is not necessarily limited by growing older or aging.

Getting back to the Tasaday, they're very loving with each other and have a very unselfconscious attitude toward sex. They treat it as a necessary body function, but one that's wrapped up in love.

The Tasaday culture, very much like the Chinese, always has venerated age, which brings with it wisdom. Our culture venerates only youth. It seems ridiculous because teenagery is such a fleeting moment in our lives (and a time when we made such asses of ourselves—at least I know *I* did!), whereas maturity and wisdom are lasting. But I firmly believe that maturity and wisdom don't have to be accompanied by a wizened, old, tired body. That's the point of this book. Think how terrific it can be to be wise and mature and still look luscious and healthy and feel full of energy. This is not only possible, it *has* to happen as night follows day if you work at it. You work at making a buck—why not work at making energy (much more important than money).

I've always heard that Chinese men make the best lovers, but I never heard the rest of the story, *why* they make the best lovers, so I did some research. I found that the Chinese culture has always advocated that young men be taught not to ejaculate, but to hold back for their own pleasure as well as for their mates'. They teach that the greatest mutual pleasure in sex comes from stimulating the female's orgasms. Men are trained to hold back as long as they can so that when they do finally have orgasms, they will be more than mere ejaculations; they will be ecstatic releases of prolonged tension.

Many doctors believe that a full male orgasm never happens without training. A man can teach himself to slow down when he thinks he will come, and the pleasure of bringing his partner to climax several times while he enjoys the sensual delights of being teased cannot be surpassed by mere ejaculation. And any woman fortunate enough to have such an enlightened mate will be the happiest woman in the world.

Teasing is the secret to great sex, and only someone who loves will take the time to tease. A real lover isn't interested in "slam, bam, thank you ma'am" or "buzz, whirr, thank you sir." That's for desperate people, people who are afraid of love or those who don't think they deserve it. Teasing is fun, like playing a game, and it builds up desire till you think you'll go crazy with it—and *that* is great sex, the unbearable desire for someone you love to pleasure you.

A woman must be coaxed into having an orgasm—and in my opinion the reason so many women have trouble climaxing is because their partner "bangs" them, which anesthetizes the clitoris and numbs all feeling, and the woman wishes the man would hurry up and get it over with. But when a man teases his love slowly and softly until her desire for him overpowers her, she will have an orgasm that will open up her very soul and send rockets and fireworks through her whole body. Sex should never be rushed; but even when you don't have a lot of time on your hands, making love should be just that—doing loving, gentle things to each other to turn each other on with delicious feeling.

Dr. Eugene Scheimann, in his book *Sex Can Save Your Heart and Life*, says that sexual pleasure can bring harmony and happiness into our lives—and it can also make us physically healthier. He says:

1. Sex is the best and cheapest remedy for emotional stress.
2. Sex is excellent exercise and effective therapy.
3. Sex helps prevent hormone imbalance and reduces the narrowing of coronary arteries.
4. Sex can reduce the cholesterol level.
5. Sex helps ease the frustrations of "coronary risks" who are then less likely to eat, drink or smoke to excess.
6. Sex often assures a happier, more harmonious family life. Heart attack is 50% more frequent among unmarried men.
7. Sex for men in the later years prevents the false "menopausal syndrome," masculinity crisis and impotency.
8. Sex for women satisfies basic needs—and sex can slow down the aging process.
9. Sex invites tenderness and togetherness and discourages, hostility, self-destruction and loneliness.
10. Sex and love provide hope, optimism and a positive state of mind and well-being—crucial factors in the treatment of heart and other stress-related diseases.

Love is more out in the open now, and being affectionate is fun. You can't be lovey-dovey if you're all tensed up by mental tension (where am I going to get the money to pay all these bills?) emotional tension (I don't think she really cares—else why was she so turned on by that guy at the party?) and physical tension (I feel like I'm going to jump right out of my skin).

So once you take care of the physical with the yeast, lecithin, and vites, the mental and emotional will calm down too—remember they all work synergistically, or together—and even though the yeast, lecithin, and vites won't bring the money to pay the bills, they will relax you so much that all that trapped energy wasted in tension will be released so you can figure out in a relaxed state where you'll get the money or how you can stall gracefully till you can lay your hands on some cash. And now that you're not so tense physically, maybe you'll pat your roomie, wife, or husby lovingly on the behind to show affectionately that you care.

In Gail Sheehy's book *Predictable Crises of Adult Life,* she tells of a man who, during his thirties as a divorced man, was a stud-about-town. Then, when he was almost forty and happily remarried, his wife went out of town on business, and a playmate from his past asked him to a party. After the party they went to bed, but he couldn't get an erection, which disturbed him immensely. And the next few times with other women, he still couldn't get it up. He finally figured out that besides feeling guilty for lying to his wife, he felt that he was being used by these other women. The sex had no emotion or feelings attached to it—it was just sex for sex's sake. He couldn't perform on demand. Finally he realized the advantage to wanting affection and exclusivity with sex rather than using sex for dominance He saw that he had gained the freedom not to have to chase after women, and he became more attached to and more in love with his wife.

Ever since the flower children of the '60s expressed love unselfconsciously, people seem to be less afraid of showing affection. We're in the Age of Aquarius now, and that's a time for caring more about humanity.

And sex—sex is definitely out of the closet. More and more people are beginning to realize that sex expression isn't dirty but is a sign of a healthy appetite, just like a hearty appetite for food is a sign of good health. When a person or an animal is sick, the last thing they want is food. A loss of appetite is a sure sign of bodily or emotional malfunction. If you're repressed emotionally, it will show itself in a tense, uptight body. And then again, a tense, uptight body will house repressed emotions. You can't have one without the other. Tension is the enemy of energy. The body, mind, and emotions function as one unit, and if one part isn't functioning it will affect the others. So if sex isn't pleasurable to you, or you're afraid of it, or if it seems "dirty" to you, first clear up your physical body. Stop putting junk into your personal machine and start putting in the right nutrients.

A friend of mine, a much older but energetic man who was a tycoon in radio and is now into other fields, told me how he got into nutrition. He bought a country club and golf course in New Jersey about twenty-five years ago, and the lawn was turning brown and looked awful. He called in a gardener who advised giving the lawn vitamins (he called fertilizer vitamins, which of course it really is) and when my friend watched the brown, ugly lawn turn to lush green, he saw what vites could do for grass and started taking them himself—and he's incredibly young for his age. I asked a few of his girl friends about his S.Q., and they all said the vites work!

Apropos of sex, I'd like to bring in cigarette smoking again. Dr. Alton Ochsner, M.D., is a senior consultant to the Ochsner Foundation Hospital in New Orleans, and twenty-eight years before the surgeon general's report on smoking came out, Dr. Ochsner found a cause-and-effect relationship between heavy cigarette smoking and lung cancer, based on observing many patients. He is convinced by the same kind of clinical evidence that cigarette smoking is dangerous to one's sexual health. He says it's much easier to get his patients to stop smoking when they believe it will help their sex lives rather than their lungs or hearts.

Dr. Joel Fort, M.D., director of the Center for Solving Special Social and Health Problems in San Francisco, which helps people to deal with sexual problems and to kick the cigarette habit, tells smokers who have impotence problems to enroll in the center's clinic to stop smoking. Almost all of the men who do so report that their sex lives improve considerably. And women who had no interest in sex perked up markedly after they gave up smoking.

Smoking impairs sexual performance in two ways—the nicotine intake constricts the blood vessels, the swelling of which is the central mechanism of sexual excitement and erection in both men and women; and the carbon monoxide intake reduces the blood oxygen level and impairs

65

hormone production. The secondary effect of heavy smoking is that lung capacity is reduced, cutting back on stamina and the ability to last during intercourse.

Two French researchers, Dr. H. Cendron and J. Vallery-Masson, published a study of the effects of age, tobacco, and other factors on male sexual activity. They took seventy men, forty-five to ninety years old, and divided them into two groups—thirty-one who smoked one or more packs a day, and thirty-nine who either were non-smokers or consumed fewer than five cigarettes a day. A little more than half the men had reported a decline in sexual activity between the ages of twenty-five and forty. There was a considerable difference between the smokers and nonsmokers—sexual activity between ages twenty-five and forty decreased more often in the first group than in the second group.

If you're short of breath and tired from smoking too much, you won't feel too much like making love—but if you stop smoking, start eating right, and begin to exercise a little, your sexual interest and ability will vastly improve.

Dr. Ochsner hopes that today's awareness of sex will cause more scientific interest in studying the effects of smoking on sexual response. Many men and women don't recognize they have a libido problem until after they've quit smoking, and then they become aware of what they've been missing.

When you get your personal machine in great working condition, I guarantee that your sexual appetite will become healthy and many emotional repressions will leave.

Making love with someone you care for isn't "dirty" any more than is eating a luscious apple. Sex is merely the release of tension in your body. We're made up of many chemicals and electrical impulses. When we go too long without sexual release, our bodies get very tense and nervous, and eventually in our sleep we may have a very pleasant dream and wake up feeling better. So one way or the other nature wins out.

Certain athletes flaunt their sex-before-games in spite of their coaches' warnings that it drains them of energy. Joe Namath, right after winning the 1969 Jets–Baltimore Colts Super Bowl game, publicly told television and radio and newspaper reporters how the night before playing he'd had sex and it made him play better. Also Derek Sanderson doesn't believe in the no-sex thing before games. When he plays for the Boston Bruins in the rough, tough body contact sport of hockey, he likes plenty of body contact before a game.

Walter Cronkite says that sex is very important in his life and that a healthy sex life is a great aid to being well adjusted.

Arlene Dahl says sex is the number one beauty treatment for women—and thank God something so good is good for us. If every woman had her attitude, there would be a lot more relaxed, loving faces and bodies around—male and female.

Now, lots of people need a drink before they can do anything, including making love—they feel it loosens them up. But if your body is loaded with yeast and vites, you'll be relaxed all the time. All that ugly tension you're used to feeling in your body will disappear, and a fantastic feeling of well-being will take over. People drink because they're afraid—they may not consciously realize they're afraid, but fear is in the head because tension is in the body.

As I pointed out before, tension is trapped energy, and once you untrap it, all the released energy will make your body feel supergood. Experiments have proved that if the body is perfectly relaxed, a person cannot experience negative emotions. That's the basic theory behind sodium pentathol (truth serum). It makes your muscles so relaxed that you're not afraid to tell the truth. Perfect relaxation gets rid of jealousy, insecurity, hatred, fear, and replaces them with love and a sense of well-being. That's another thing the yeast and dolomite tablets will do for you—make you relaxed in a healthy way so you won't need alcohol to relax you in an unhealthy way. Of course one or two drinks aren't going to hurt anyone—I'm only talking about the extreme category, into which so many people fall.

Alcoholism is mostly a physical problem—if you cure your body's chemical imbalance with yeast and vites, you will find the craving for alcohol has left. Dr. Roger J. Williams and other scientists have shown that nutritional deficiencies cause the desire to drink.

Polly Bergen is a beautiful actress, singer, and businesswoman, and it took a traumatic divorce for her to find her real self and to write a book about it so she could help other women with emotional and sexual problems like the ones she had had before her reawakening. Her book is

Polly's Principles, and in it she tells how her sexual inhibitions were a large part of the ruination of her marriage. She says that sex and beauty cannot be separated, and that sex is second only to love as a beauty treatment. Polly says you must force yourself to be unselfconscious about your body, and this goes for men as well as women (not all men are uninhibited—in fact, many aren't). It's amazing how people change and times change. A few years ago people weren't as outspoken about sex as they are now, and frankness is a real step in the right direction.

Virginia Graham has a wonderful feeling about sex—"the completion of a circle of emotional fulfillment and a natural function of the body." She believes all the inhibitions have been taught by parents and the churches. But just as any extreme is unhealthy—too much food or too little sleep—and discipline is necessary in every facet of life, sexual discipline is vital for the emotional health of the community. But as Virginia points out, sex must be functioning before it can be disciplined.

Sheila MacRae feels that sex is a natural outcome of wanting to get out of yourself and experience what the other person is like, and that way you find yourself.

Psychologist Joyce Brothers says that today's kids are rejecting the detached, uncommitted sex that was thriving during the sexual revolution of the flower children and psychedelic drugs; that today they're more loving in their sexual relationships, and both boys and girls want more commitment.

Dr. Masters of Masters and Johnson avers that commitment and a strong emotional tie make a sexual relationship "infinitely more effective."

Chryssa Dobson, a writer for *Cosmopolitan* magazine, makes a terrific case for sex with love as opposed to a different lover every day.

> Really good sex comes only when you grow sensitive enough to another person to know what pleases him or her both in and out of bed . . . a skill hardly likely to develop overnight. You can't learn to play a musical instrument in a day; what horror to imagine trying to learn a *different* musical instrument each afternoon.

So when you're living with or around someone you truly love, sex is a beautiful way to express that love.

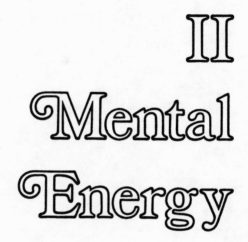

II
Mental
Energy

4
SELF-HYPNOSIS: IF IT CAN TAKE AWAY PAIN, IT CAN PUT IN HAPPINESS

And it will if you use it. We don't realize it, but we've all been programmed or hypnotized into the beliefs we carry with us today. If we're successful, we carry an image of ourselves as deserving success, and if we're not, we carry self-images of failure and doubt. When we were kids we were either programmed by our parents or our teachers or our pals or ourselves into believing we were certain types of people. If you constantly heard what a dumbbell you were, eventually you believed it and have subconsciously believed it all your life. No matter how hard you try, underneath that smiling face is a dumbbell self-image.

What has to be done is reprogramming or re-self-hypnosis. The self-image must be changed to one of a terrific person—kind, bright, thoughtful of others, fun-loving—a mensch, as they say. And why not? Who among us isn't capable of doing *something* well? No one is a genius in all areas, and no one is a klutz in all areas. Every one of us has some area where he or she can shine. Auto-suggestion can completely change your life.

Phyllis Diller used self-hypnosis and developed a tremendous belief in herself. Walter Cronkite used self-hypnosis to change his caring about competition—he now doesn't give a hoot about the ratings of his competitors. He competes with himself—he's only interested if he's doing his best. Autosuggestion can be used by every one of us to make our lives happier.

Jim Bouton totally believes that self-hypnosis has changed his life, and he says he'll never stop using it.

He was just another pitcher for the New York Yankees —but he was a cut above the average player. He was a very colorful and expressive guy. Had he just remained a ballplayer, the world wouldn't have known about him. But he wrote a book, *Ball Four*, which exposed the baseball heroes with all their foibles—he showed them with their gloves off. As a result, he made a few enemies and changed his career. He's now one of the very few TV sports commentators with a sense of humor—he's a very whimsical guy.

Jim is one who understands and practices self-hypnosis and has seen many other people benefit from it. He has total concentration. Many times after pitching a winning game he would walk off the mound and not remember one thing that happened. He has the ability to sweep his mind clear of everything but the job before him and concentrate totally on one thing. When he went to Hollywood to do his first film, he used his concentration to bring in a good performance. Of course all actors use self-hypnosis and concentration to do their parts, but the real point is that every human being uses self-hypnosis unconsciously and doesn't even know it.

A coach once told Jim when he was nervous before a game to just remember that 600 million Chinese don't give a damn whether he wins or loses, so he shouldn't make it life or death—just relax and do his best. And it worked. Jim used the mental image of his game being so unimportant to the rest of the world that his importance dwindled too, and pitching became easier—less a matter of life and death.

When you go out to do something, you either believe you can, or you accept the belief that you really can't do it. For instance, if you go out for a job interview, either you believe you can do it and should get the job, or not. The more you believe you can do it, the more positive self-hypnosis you are using; but the more you believe you can't do it, the more negative self-hypnosis you are using.

People generally think of hypnosis as only a trancelike state where one person has control over another. But that's not true. Hypnosis is a direct line of communication from the conscious to the subconscious mind, which is a vast reservoir of power and is generally untapped by most of us. All a hypnotist does is tap the subconscious mind to get us to do so-called superhuman feats. If our subconscious is told we have twice the strength that our conscious minds believe we have, and if our subconscious believes this to be absolutely true, then our bodies will act as if we are twice as strong as we previously thought.

Now if an outsider can reach our subconscious, so can we. There's a knack and an art to doing it, but it's really worth practicing. We can program our subconscious to accept anything we want it to. We can tell our subconscious we want to be smarter, and once our subconscious accepts this we will release hidden powers of intelligence we never knew we had. Just as we were programmed as kids by all the adults around us and we more or less accepted their opinions of us, we can now change it by the same means— repetition of belief.

If I keep telling myself what a disciplined person I am, and I do this with feeling because it's *important* to me to be disciplined, my subconscious will soon accept this and I will *be* more disciplined. It can become easier and easier for me to lose weight, because my subconscious will take over the job and food will become less and less important. If I keep telling myself I want to become very successful and make a lot of money, my subconscious will lead me to opportunities that I never would have thought of had I just been working with my conscious mind (or forebrain thinking, as it's called).

You'll never know till you put this to the test what incredible things your own subconscious can and will do for you if you only learn how to tap its power. It's like a sleeping giant just waiting for you to wake it up. It's the source of your whole future. But unfortunately most of us just let our subconscious be led by the beliefs fed into it when we were being programmed. As kids we just accepted what mummy and daddy and teacher thought of us. Today if someone doesn't like us or is negative, we can tune out and not accept this opinion. As kids we accepted everything; after all, what did we know about ourselves or life around us? It takes experience to teach us to sift through thoughts and take the positive and reject the negative.

So if you've been carrying around lots of negatives through your life—and which of us couldn't get rid of *some* negative thought we picked up as kids?—now's the time to clear out the conscious mind (and you do this by just hanging on to positive thoughts and not allowing any negatives in) and contact the subconscious mind.

Emmet Fox wrote *Power through Constructive Thinking*, and in the book he has a chapter entitled "The Seven Day Mental Diet" in which he states that the food with which you furnish your mind determines the total character of your life. Just as your whole body is really composed of the food you have eaten in the past—the food you eat today will be in your bloodstream after a few hours, and your bloodstream builds all the tissues making up your body—the thoughts that you feed your mind, the mental diet on which you live, make you and your surroundings what they are. He calls it the Great Cosmic Law and says that if you change your mind and your thoughts, your conditions must change also.

A few years ago I went on the seven-day mental diet, and it was the toughest thing I've ever done. Giving up food is much easier than giving up thoughts we're used to, even though they're negative. I stuck it out for the seven days, and my life definitely changed, slowly at first, but absolutely in a positive direction.

When you begin the diet, all kinds of thoughts seem to be stirred up and negatives fly at you from all directions, but that's a good sign. Your whole world of thought is moving and changing and rocking, but you just hang on, and when the moving and changing and rocking is over, your mental picture and actual life will have reassembled itself into something much closer to what you want.

It was a beginning point of a new way of thinking for me. In looking back, I most remember three things for having worked changes for the better in my life. The first was reading Ralph Waldo Emerson. His essays, "Self Reliance," "The Oversoul," "Compensation," "Spiritual Laws," "Love," "Friendship," "Circles," "Intellect," and many more (I read every essay many times and they're all great) changed my mind and my path of life. From a dopey, confused, religious, high school girl, I became a person who began to think for herself. (I'm actually much *more* religious now, with a feeling for good and love, than I was then, with my cerebral concept of God that was pounded into me from the first grade through graduation in my senior year.)

The second mental milestone was a quote I read in Bob Cummings's book, *Stay Young and Vital:* "A great burden falls away if we let God run the universe."

I so clearly remember putting the book down and taking a long walk with my dog and thinking about that sentence. Up till then *I* was running the universe—and I was a nervous wreck. Suddenly I saw my pitiful, weak little self struggling to run my universe and how ridiculous it was. All that the struggle brought was enormous tension as I tried to force things to happen. I discovered that all a person can do is his or her best and then allow things to happen if they're meant to be.

The third big change came about after completing the seven-day mental diet. It literally changed my way of thinking and doing. but as I mentioned before, it's the toughest thing I've ever done—even tougher than cutting out smokes, and *that* was tough for me.

During the mental diet I worked my imagination overtime. I pictured myself hanging onto a huge rock which was the only steady thing in the center of my quaking world of negatives as my little world shook violently. But I hung on for dear life. Every time a negative thought tried to enter my mind, I thought of it as a cigarette ash which I immediately flicked off (if an ash stays even a second, it burns). So between flicking off negatives and hanging on to my giant rock while my whole world shook all around me, I was kept very busy policing the thoughts trying to enter my mind. And of course, the more you try *not* to think negatively, the more these kinds of thoughts are conjured up, so not letting them enter was some kind of job. It was as if every negative in my whole life became aware of my struggle and tried to defeat me, and this made it sort of exciting. If it were easy, it wouldn't have given me such a great feeling of accomplishment. If you think it's easy, just try it for an hour, much less seven days. It takes someone who wants to change his or her life from negative to positive—someone very determined—and anyone reading this book is a self-helper (who better to help?) and can do the mental diet.

When I finished it, my way of thinking definitely had changed. Unconscious negatives ("I won't get that part I read for in the TV show," "They promised to pay me by Friday, but I know they won't and I'm going to be late with the rent again") stopped bugging me—in fact, my mind was a lot clearer. It had to be when the junky negs were cleared out and the positives could work. It's just like a computer—you have to clear out all the mistakes before it can work properly—and the human brain is the same.

Thinking positively will get rid of compulsive thoughts and tormenting fears that many people can't get rid of except by blunting or dulling them through tranquilizers, booze, or mind-changing drugs. People who successfully complete the seven-day mental diet (not less than seven days), will have proved to themselves that *they* are in control of their thoughts and that all thoughts must obey a personal command. Their thoughts will become slaves to their will, and they will have a feeling of mental power that they never had before.

It's not the thoughts that enter your mind that matter, only those that you choose to dwell upon that count. You yourself are active in choosing what you want to think about. You can continue thinking negatively and go on in the same negative rut, complaining about how you're a victim of life, or you can actively do something about changing your whole outlook and, inevitably, your whole life.

A terrific way to make contact with your subconscious is to stand in front of a mirror and stare into your eyes and talk aloud to yourself. Tell yourself exactly what you want out of life. One of the very saddest things we're taught is that we shouldn't want much from life, to expect pain and suffering and not to expect good things to happen. That's one of the worst things that most churches teach: that God is vindictive, when we do bad we will be punished, and "bad" is generally doing what gives us pleasure—so most of us expect to be punished for pleasure, and to get defeated in our quest for the good life. And it's a vicious circle because nature wants us pleasured and tempts us with the good things of life. Then when we experience these wonderful natural things, our preprogrammed guilt takes over and makes us miserable.

But the truth of the matter is that the subconscious mind, as lots of people are beginning to understand, is impersonally and objectively waiting for us to program into it only positive thoughts and only positive results will happen. Our subconscious is not a moral judge interested in how "good" or "bad" we are; it's just there, waiting for us to contact it. Lots of so-called atheists say they don't believe in any God—they only believe in mind power. But can't mind power be God? Some of us need to see God as a personalized father-figure, and others need to see the impersonality of God. But that Spirit, or Life-Force, or whatever you want to call it, still exists, no matter in what form we prefer to accept or reject it.

If you really wish to do something, get your subconscious to do it for you. If you really want to stop smoking because you know how awful it is for your body, get your subconscious mind to do all the work. Stand in front of a mirror and tell yourself you are quitting cigarettes. Every chance you get, look into a mirror and tell yourself the same thing and explain to yourself that every cell in your body is going to get really healthy. And when you're not around a mirror, visualize your face and repeat your desire. Before you fall asleep, tell yourself you're quitting. When you wake up in the morning, repeat your desire. You will reprogram your thinking and without realizing it you will soon lose your desire for a ciggie. This is self-hypnosis, and it really works. And you can use it for losing weight or gaining a new girl friend (or boyfriend).

But just as the positive works, so does the negative. If you keep repeating downers about yourself and others

—like "I always catch colds" and "People are all out to get me"—you're hypnotizing yourself into accepting these negatives.

Why not use this enormous power to do something or get something that will make you happy? If you want money, close your eyes and visualize all the things you'd like to buy—a gorgeous wardrobe, a groovy car, a fantastic apartment, a month in the Bahamas, a yacht—go all the way. When you do your mirror work, tell yourself exactly what you want. Start with the wardrobe (if that's what you want first), look right into your eyes, and tell yourself you want your subconscious to get it for you. Those of you who don't think I'm completely bananas and who really try this will get what you want.

A relaxed, tension-free body, bursting with constructive energy, will house a much more positive, relaxed mind, and it will be much easier to reprogram positive attitudes into that mind when you've filled your body with yeast and vites. Nothing is all physical or all mental—we're a combination of physical, mental, and emotional—but the first one to start healing is the physical, because it's the house in which the other two reside. Once you get the body in great shape, you'll find you'll automatically be more positive and working with the subconscious will become not only easier, but the natural thing for you to do.

Time magazine recently ran a paragraph on Shirley MacLaine and what she had to say shows how aware she is of herself and how constructive that is:

Backed by a big band for her first show at the London Palladium, actress Shirley MacLaine showed few of her 41 years. "My muscles are better, my breathing is better, and that's because I'm more relaxed," said she. "When you know who you are and you realize what you can do, you can do things better at 40 than when you're 20."

Bing Crosby was reborn in 1935 on the "Kraft Music Hall." Up until that time, in the late '20s and early '30s, he couldn't say hello without a script. He had no identity. He was a complete introvert who could only express himself through singing, so he turned to alcohol to loosen himself up, and eventually he was dependent on it. Then he met Cal Kuhl and Carroll Carroll, two writers on the Kraft Music Hall, and they wrote a complete personality for him—a droll, slow-talking, humorous ad-libber—and he became that personality. Suddenly he had an identity, and one that he dug. His confusion was over, and his newfound personality was an instant hit. People liked him; and better yet, *he* liked him.

Identity-confusion is one of the biggest psychological reasons for someone drinking, explaining why so many homosexuals, male and female, are alcoholics—they don't know if they want to be men or women, a pretty basic confusion.

But once they make their decision to either come out of the closet and admit to homosexuality and live as happy a life as possible, or to try, through therapy, to accept the sex they were physically born with, the drinking problem leaves.

Any confusion is debilitating. It's pitting self against self, where both lose.

George Balanchine, the brilliant ballet-choreographer now in his seventies, was asked how it happens that he's more vigorous now than when he was younger. He replied: "I've got more energy now than when I was young because I know exactly what I want to do." He believes that younger people are usually more confused than the older, more mature person. Until we find out what we want —what we *really* want—out of life, we can't use self-hypnosis to go after it. So a major step in everyone's life is to consciously make an effort to find out where our talents lie.

A very intelligent approach to this, in my opinion, is to take an aptitude test, or several aptitude tests. Every city has places where they're given. Call the public library in your city and ask for help in locating where you can take the test. At least it will work as a guide to show you areas of complete ineptness and areas of no natural inclination, and at most it will uncover hidden talents you never knew you possessed. For instance, you might find that colors are important to you, that you've a creative nature, and that you should work indoors, so you decide to quit driving a truck and you enroll in a school for interior design. Or you may find that children stimulate you and that you have a very sympathetic nature and want to help others, so you begin working with retarded kids and are truly happy and fulfilled for the first time in your life. It's amazing how little we know ourselves, and what better *should* we know? But once the decision is made and you truly know where you want to go in the exciting adventure of life, you can really begin to use your subconscious and make all your wildest dreams come true.

All of Alex Cohen's wildest dreams came true. He started out as a young, twenty-one-year-old angel and co-producer of a smash hit, *Angel Street*, which made a lot of money for him. Right after that he went into public relations for Bulova watches, and dreamed up some super publicity stunts, but he couldn't stay away from Broadway. He became a producer of a string of flops, but undaunted, he finally came up with *At the Drop of a Hat*, the first of nine successive hits, such as *An Evening with Mike Nichols and Elaine May, Beyond the Fringe*, and *Maurice Chevalier at 77*. Now he's always got some hit on Broadway, and he's the television producer of the spectacular Tony Awards, put on every year on national TV. Alex practices self-hypnosis and has hypnotized himself over a period of years. He says it's the most powerful force in his life, and if everyone would realize the power of the sub-conscious, everyone would be a success.

Sheila MacRae uses self-hypnosis before any stage or television performance. An hour before she's due on stage, she gets by herself and mentally and psychically focuses all her energy on one thing—success. She never thinks of the audience. She pulls all her thoughts in and con-centrates solely on doing a good job. She has developed her concentration over the years so that she's able to shut everything else out but positive thoughts of success. Sheila calls this "moment-to-moment thinking."

She also controls her body through self-hypnosis. She keeps her weight down and her body trim by mastering her mind and thoughts. It must work, 'cause she looks great!

Sammy Cahn says he feels better at sixty-one than ever before, and he talks to himself a lot (which is basically self-hypnosis). He says that when he is confronted with any problem, he asks himself what is the natural law of it, and the logical answer comes to him.

Hildegarde says she uses self-hypnosis a lot and that it's pulled her through a lot of trying situations. She feels that the power of your subconscious is enormous and it's a pity more people aren't aware of it. She suggests a book by Dr. Joseph Murphy called *The Power of Your Subconscious Mind*, which I plan on reading as soon as I finish this book.

Arlene Dahl constantly uses self-hypnosis and says you can do what you think and believe you can do. Because she's aware of this, she uses her subconscious every day.

When we can see that self-hypnosis is not a spooky, mystical, "you are falling under my spell, you are going into a trance" kind of thing, but a harnessing of our all-powerful subconscious minds (our Giant Selves), and using this power for obtaining everything we want out of life, that's when we will know real happiness and fulfillment. If we use self-hypnosis to raise our self-confidence and to really begin to believe in ourselves, we will release the tensions of self-doubt and fear of failing, and these tensions (trapped energy) will be released and the released energy will enable us to go after what we want and get it!

5
THE KNOCKERS VERSUS THE DOERS

There are doers and there are knockers. The doers aren't afraid of failing (or if they are they overcome it) and are busy trying to accomplish. The knockers are the critics of the world. They sit back and judge everything —nothing is spared. When they taste a wine, it's not as good as it might have been. When they see a play, it's not as good as it might have been. *Nothing* is as good as it might have been. It's sad, because only those who don't do, knock.

Look around you and listen. The real doers never knock. And the nondoers use knocking as an excuse not to do. They're too busy putting everything down—every little detail—and feeling so important as a critic that they're let off their own hook (they feel no guilt) for not doing. It takes time and energy to be a critic—but it's wasted, negative energy—and it will get you nothing. It's a passive way of kidding yourself into thinking you're doing. There are ways to become a participator instead of just sitting on the sidelines of life pretending to be the authority on everything.

Of all kinds of criticism, self-criticism is the worst. Most good actors are too self-critical. When I did a lead on a "Bonanza" with the late Dan Blocker—he was Hoss and I was Big Red—I found out he was always critical of his performance, always trying to do better. Usually this is good, but when a performance is already terrific and a guy still frets, it can be destructive. And Don Rickles, whom I worked with on a TV show, was his own worst critic and had to change his way of thinking and accept himself so that he became a good actor besides being a funny man.

One of the most draining and enervating of all self-criticisms is regret. To regret having done anything is self-defeating. "Why did I tell him that? I never should have opened my mouth." "Why did I pick this job instead of that other, terrific one? What a fool I was." The only foolishness is allowing this kind of thinking. It's illogical and dumb. At the time we make decisions, we weigh everything and do what we think is best. Later on, if it doesn't turn out so hot, we castigate ourselves. Dumb.

We did what we had to do at that time. If we had been able to make another decision, we would have. Think back. Transport yourself mentally back to the time of a decision. You weighed both sides and finally decided on one course of action. Had you thought the other was better, you would have done it, and if you were confused, you chose what you thought at the time was the better of the two ways. It's easy to Monday-morning-quarterback, but it's dumb. We can and should learn from our mistakes, but sometimes our mistakes are not really mistakes, but a link in a chain of happenings that couldn't have happened without the so-called mistake.

I'm a complete fatalist because to me it's the most logical outlook of all. But by fatalism I do not mean a passive waiting for things to happen. I mean an active use of our intelligence to go after what we want—and then, after we have done our very best, to relax and know that *che será, será*—what will be, will be. In other words, after doing our best, we should let things happen and not try to force them.

If you look back objectively on your life you'll see that most of the events which happened weren't caused by you at all, but because another person did something or an event happened that changed your whole life without your lifting a finger. I can remember when I first went to Buenos Aires, and every night I'd walk down a certain street to go to the downtown area to eat dinner. One evening, for no apparent reason, I decided to take another avenue and I bumped into a producer I had met in Caracas a few months earlier. We stopped in a confiteria for coffee and made a deal for me to star in an American film to be shot there. Had I not walked down that particular street that particular night, I wouldn't have met the producer, and my whole life would have been different.

It was fate. It was meant to be and it really was not my doing—a higher self (again the subconscious, which I call my Giant Self) led me to the other street. It was not through my own will; and in reality, very few things happen because we make them. Most things happen circumstantially. Look at your own life. Think back. Either you met someone and your life changed (so you didn't really *do* anything—something was done *to* you) or maybe you fell and broke a leg, and because you were forced into bed rest you had a lot of time to think and you decided on a complete new course of your life (which never would have happened without the accident). As my all-time favorite philosopher, Ralph Waldo Emerson, said:

> What has my will done to make me that I am? Nothing. I have been floated into this thought, this hour, this connection of events, by secret currents of might and mind, and my ingenuity and willfulness have not thwarted, have not aided, to an appreciable degree.

So if you can logically see how fate works in your life, you can logically see how dumb it is to regret anything. It happened because it *had* to happen, it was meant to happen; so learn from it, forget it, and go on and use the energy you'll get from dropping what you *don't* want to go after what you *do* want.

Some people point out that fatalism is foolish because all you have to do is sit back and wait for things to happen. But that's not fatalism, that's stupidity. True fatalism says do the best you can and *then* know that what will be, will be. Do your best job, then relax and don't fight fate. And of course, never ever regret anything you've ever done, no matter how foolish it seems in retrospect. At that time when you did it, you *had* to do it or else you would have done something different. If you said something which now appears to be stupid and you lost a deal or a friend and they can't be salvaged, know that on the path your subconscious is leading you, it's better that you lost the deal or the friend. It's meant to be that you go along another path, and there will be other, better deals and other, better friends.

The other side of the coin is guilt. Castigating yourself for having done something which you consciously or unconsciously think is wrong, or "bad," is wasted energy. You have two choices—if you still believe what you've done is bad or wrong, resolve to never do it again and then forget it. I mean purge it out of your mind and replace it with the thought of a constructive action—or analyze what you've done in the cold light of today—bring yourself up to date—forget what mummy or daddy or teacher said years ago, and realize you're no longer a little kid. Just analyze your action and see if it's really so awful. Did you hurt yourself? Did you hurt someone else? If so, realize that that was a phase of your life that you had to go through, that was an experience you had to know, and your subconscious had you do it for a reason. Everything that happens in life is for a reason. If you can understand it, good. If not, you can try to develop a belief that everything works out for the best, that even the things that don't appear to be for the best, in the long-range plan of life will be constructive.

Happy people are doers—activists, not passive onlookers.

Lots of entertainers refuse to read critiques of their performances. If they believe the raves, they've got to believe the pans—and maybe the critic had a fight with his wife that morning or has a terrific hangover and can't wait to get out of the show and get a drink, or doesn't like tall, thin men (they remind him of his father). A couple of years ago I clipped out of two magazines two reviews of a Shirley MacLaine movie. One critic, a woman, thought it was one of the best films of the last ten years, and the other critic, a man, nominated it for one of the year's ten worst films. It was incredible. Two intelligent people, two of the top critics, with diametrically opposed opinions; and yet if you read one you'd rush right out to see this work of art, but if you read the other you'd tell all your acquaintances that this is one film they didn't release—it escaped.

Jeffrey Lyons, film and theater critic on CBS Radio and WPIX-TV, is a New York critic and a very good one.

I could be accused of being biased in thinking he's a good critic because he gave *Be Kind to People Week*, the Off-Broadway show I starred in this year, a good review, but then so did a few others; so my respect for Jeffrey is only because he truly tries to give an objective analysis of what he's watching.

The night before he became a critic a few years ago, he had dinner at Sardi's with the wonderful and beautiful Ruth Gordon (can you ever forget her fantastically fey performance in *Harold and Maude*?) and she told him, "Think twice before you shit on somebody else's work"; and I believe Jeffrey always has (thought twice, that is).

He analyzes more than criticizes, and that's constructive rather than destructive (as opposed to some critics who try to be funny at the expense of whatever is being reviewed—like the critic who reviewed *I Am a Camera* many years ago on Broadway; one can imagine his eagerness to hate the show so he could use his clever two-word review, "No Leica." P.S., the show was a huge hit).

Analysis is fine to cull the wheat from the chaff, but after that, criticism can get in the way of action. Excessive criticism is negative, and anything negative stops progress and energy. One of the most negative things that keeps people from accomplishing what they desire is the fear of failing, and this comes from self-criticism. We all tend to think other people's accomplishments are grand and our own are miniscule. It always seems that other people accomplish things easily—without sweat and hard work. But when *we* do something, it's pure drudgery. "Why do

I have to work so hard when he gets it so easily?" Nonsense. Hard work is the answer to *all* accomplishment. And those who do accomplish push fear of failure out of their minds. After all, what's the worst thing that can happen? You fail. That doesn't mean you're a failure. You failed at one thing—big deal! Anyone who's ever tried to do *anything* has failed, and probably many times. But that still doesn't make you a failure. The only thing that can do that is your own attitude, and once you stop criticizing yourself and those around you, your attitude will automatically change from a fear of failing to a love of doing.

Henry Ford, the Detroit automaker and genius of automobile design, didn't believe in veneration of the past or fear of the future—and especially fear of failure. He said, "Failure is only the opportunity more intelligently to begin again. There is no disgrace in honest failure; there is disgrace in fearing to fail."

Johnny Carson is not at all competitive with other people—he's only concerned that he's improving his work—that each show is better than the last. He doesn't care about criticism or whether he's better than other comedians or talk-show hosts. He concentrates his energies on doing his best and making his best better and better.

Sid Caesar is just the opposite. He's very unsure of himself and the least criticism can upset him. He's worried that maybe the stagehands don't like him. This is not to say he's any less talented than other comedians—he's one of the most brilliantly funny men who ever lived. (Can you ever forget the ten-minute skit from "Your Show of

Shows" where he stands alone in a room dressing? First he puts on the military pants . . . then the jacket with the epaulettes which he polishes . . . then the shoes, which he shines to a glow . . . down to the last piece of clothing, a military visored cap with much brass. He's a picture of military grandeur with a smirk only Sid Caesar can pull off as he looks arrogantly into the camera. Finally he walks out the door, whips a whistle out of his pocket and hails a cab for a customer—he's a doorman at a restaurant.) But Sid Caesar's ego is weak and vulnerable to others' opinions, and this can be very mentally draining on his energy.

Any influence that hurts your morale compromises your power. An ego must be built up through mental processes so that a person is above worrying over other people's opinions. Once you're sure of yourself, you'll do your best job, know it's your best job, and forget about it.

Frank Sinatra is one guy who's never looked back with regret. He says if he had it to do over again, he'd do it exactly the same way. The lyrics of his big hit song tell it perfectly, "I did it my way." Frank was a big star when he was very young in 1941 and it lasted till 1948, when he hit a decline where he stayed for a few years. He made a lot of so-called mistakes, recorded wrong songs (wrong for him), changed his management several times, had a number of emotional problems, divorced his wife, married Ava Gardner, divorced her, lost his voice, had a lot of well-publicized fights, and then made a giant comeback in *From Here to Eternity*, for which he won the Oscar. Not long after that he recorded "Young at Heart," which was his first big record hit in a long period of time. Then he went on to become one of the biggest stars of all time.

But with all the valleys between the hills, Frank never wishes he'd done anything different. He did it his way, and he's smart enough to know that that's the only way. You can listen to advice, you can weigh everything, you can ask for opinions, but the final decisions are yours; and good, bad, or indifferent, you have to live with them. And any regrets or recriminations or self-criticism are enervating. If you want to change your life, change it, but if you like where you're going, accept your mistakes as veerings a torpedo makes until it corrects itself—then it veers a little in the other direction, until finally it heads straight for the target. A torpedo is unemotional—it only knows where it's going. It doesn't get upset when it makes a "mistake," or stop itself altogether and think it's stupid for veering a little; it just keeps going to its target. And once we can get the self-doubt and self-criticism (and "other-criticism," which leads to self-criticism) out of our heads, we'll hit our targets, too.

6

IF YOU KNOW WHAT YOU WANT, HANG IN THERE AND YOU'LL GET IT

Press on—put the blinders on and full steam ahead. If your concentration is so pointed in one direction and no other thoughts intrude, that's the basic working of tuning in your subconscious, which is the "doer" part of the mechanism known as "you." Most of us want lots of things, and they're all scattered around. We don't spend too much time on one particular thing; and that's too bad, 'cause if we did—if we really blocked everything else out and concentrated on getting the one or two things we *really* want out of life—we would get them, absolutely and without question.

There are rules in the universe. If you concentrate the sun's rays through a magnifying glass on a paper. the paper will burn. And if you concentrate thought, which is more powerful than the sun's rays, on a subject, you will fire it, fan it to flames, and you will have what you want. It works; but it takes time, and most of us don't have the patience or the belief that it will work. You must never give up wanting it and thinking about it, and then your imagination comes into play.

It's been proven that when the will and the imagination are pitted against each other, the imagination always dominates. Émile Coué, the French psychologist and philosopher who lived from 1857 to 1926 and was the great advocate of autosuggestion ("every day in every way I am getting better and better"), said, "When the will and the imagination are antagonistic, it is always the imagination which wins, without any exception." To stay with imagination, mind's dominant power, Clarence Buddington Kelland, the American novelist, said:

I have been infinitely curious about people, and their whys and wherefores. I have been at some pains to study and to analyze their careers. For years I have been at it, and I believe I have discovered the one great, moving, compelling force which makes every man what he becomes in the end.

This, I believe, is the greatest force in the universe. I believe all other causes are secondary to it. It is so powerful that the slightest human effort cannot be put forth until it has done its work: and if it should suddenly be annihilated from the world, all activity would come to a standstill, and humanity would become a mass of automatons moving about sluggishly in meaningless circles.

This force is not love; it is not religion; it is not virtue; it is not ambition—for none of these could exist an hour without it. . . . It is imagination.

Every child is taught what he *should* do—but few are helped in the self-discovery of what they *can* do. What you *can* do is a call to the imagination and for action. Image-in, or put a picture in your mind of what you want. Think about it. When you want to lose weight, you can will yourself not to eat, but you'll rationalize and sneak a snack. But fall in love and start to imagine yourself as having a gorgeous body to enrapture your beloved, and your appetite will leave. Or try giving up cigarettes. Will it, and you'll struggle in vain. You'll rationalize that one little ciggie can't hurt, and you'll puff away. But let the doc tell you he gives you five more years before it's curtains, and your imagination takes over—and it's good-bye smokes. Or when you finally realize heavy smokers have very wrinkled skin and you want to keep yours loverly, there'll be no problems in stopping, unless you're a masochist who digs wrinkled skin.

But you can have the greatest imagination in the world and not be persistent enough to go after what you want, and your imagination will lead you to nothing but day-dreams.

The one quality that all successful people have that stands head and shoulders above any other qualities that they may have is persistence. They never give up. No matter what the odds in other people's minds, if it's something they really want, they just never stop working for it. In my life lots of people have said to me, "Why don't you give up on this project or that deal and go on to something new?" What most people don't realize is that they're always dropping something difficult—and everything is difficult—and going on to something new, which in turn is dropped, and so on ad infinitum. The reason there are so few successes is that most people don't stick to one thing till it's done. Naturally the stuck-to something should be important to you and worthwhile.

When I was in Chicago a couple of years ago doing television appearances, I had an idle Sunday between a Saturday and a Monday show, so I bought all the Chicago Sunday papers. In each Sunday supplement there was a full-page ad that was so terrific that I clipped them all out and brought them back to New York, and one now hangs in my apartment (another I gave to a friend as persistent as I). The ad was put in by McDonald's Hamburgers (and I don't even eat meat) and must have been suggested by the president or whoever made McDonald's the success that it is. I had visions of Irving McDonald (or whatever his name is) starting out with a teeny roadside stand selling burgers to passersby, and being told by his wife and family and all his friends that he should stop already and go back to selling insurance, but he said no—he knew he'd eventually become an American way of life. He trudged on, and his determination made him rich and famous. This is the ad:

PRESS ON

Nothing in the world can take the place of persistence. Talent will not; nothing is more common than unsuccessful men with talent. Genius will not; unrewarded genius is almost a proverb. Education alone will not; the world is full of educated derelicts. Persistence and determination alone are omnipotent.

When I decided to write this book, I decided to ask a few celebrities—mostly friends of mine—different questions about energy (all accomplishers have energy), and one of the questions was on persistence. I wanted to know exactly how determined they are.

Henny Youngman is known as the King of the One-Liners: "I've been in love with the same woman for twenty-nine years—if my wife ever finds out, she'll kill me." If he doesn't get you with his first gag, he'll get you with the second, third, or fourth. They come so fast and furious he's gotta get you sooner or later. Henny says just like he never gives up with his jokes, if he thinks he's right about wanting something, he never gives up on that, either.

Alexander Cohen, the genius-showman who has always

seen and done everything big, likes to point out he's a Leo (and he also likes to point out that Mike Todd, Billy Rose, Barnum, and Florenz Ziegfeld were Leos) and an extremely persistent person. He says of himself, "I'm a driven man."

Arlene Dahl is another Leo (and an "11"—she's into numerology and told me I'm an "11" also). She started as a showgirl at the Latin Quarter in New York, a beautiful girl with unbelievable determination. She believes she can do anything she sets her mind and heart on, and she's extremely determined to achieve what she wants. She became a movie star but wasn't content to be just another pretty face—when her movie career slowed down, she was prepared for a business life, and now she is building a cosmetics business. I've seen pictures of her when she was very young, and I think she's more beautiful today. Her determination to stay always before the public has resulted in her finding out how to keep looking gorgeous, and this is what is making her cosmetic line so successful.

David Susskind says he's unbelievably determined and persistent when he really wants something. I remember when he tried to give up smoking but couldn't. Then his doctor did a terrific thing—he took David's blood pressure and showed him the result, which was pretty normal; then he told David to smoke one cigarette, which he did. The doctor then strapped the sphygmomanometer around his arm and again took his blood pressure, which by now had jumped enormously. The doctor explained that each cigarette constricts the blood vessels in your body which causes tension and acts as an "upper." This experiment so impressed David (and his imagination) that he immediately stopped smoking and determinedly has stayed off the weed ever since. For him this takes an incredible amount of determination because he still misses smoking and says if they ever find out smoking is good for you, he's going to be first in line to buy a pack.

Jim Bouton says he's extremely tenacious. "My mother used to tell me 'You refuse to take no for an answer,' and she meant it not to be an admirable trait in a youngster; but it's meant a lot to me as I get older. I get lots more and more done."

One of the most determined people I've ever met (and charming, brilliant, clever, personable, hard-working, funny, perceptive, etc., etc., etc.) is the president of the Borough of Manhattan, Percy Sutton. He's a truly amazing man, and his persistence is remarkable. He was born in San Antonio, Texas, the son of black parents and the youngest of fifteen kids. When he was a child of seven in San Antonio, the blacks could use the public park only one day of the year. He says, "I dreamed of becoming mayor of San Antonio and one of the first things I'd do is instruct the policeman who was there to protect the bear, to permit little children of all colors to come and become entertained. At the age of seven I knew who put the policeman there, who was in charge of San Antonio, and the way to change it was to become mayor." He doesn't want to become mayor of San Antonio anymore, but I personally hope he someday becomes mayor of New York, and I do believe with his determination he'll do it!

Mark Van Doren, famous Pulitzer Prize-winning poet, believes in "being all there," or concentrating one's forces on one thing at a time and persistently holding onto the one task at hand.

> There is one thing we can do, and the happiest people are those who do it to the limit of their ability.
> We can be completely present. We can be all there. We can control the tendency of our minds to wander from the situation we are in toward yesterday, toward tomorrow, toward something we have forgotten, toward some other place we are going next. It is hard to do this, but it is harder to understand afterward wherein it was we fell so short. It was where and when we ceased to give our entire attention to the person, the opportunity, before us.

Serge Obolensky believes he's an extremely persistent person. As a child in czarist Russia, he learned discipline through sports. Every day he rode, high-jumped, rode hurdles, did lots of exercise, and today at an incredible eighty-four his posture is straight as an arrow. Colonel Obolensky was an officer in the Russian court, and after the revolution he fled to the United States where he started his life all over again in the 1920s. Today, through determination, he is running a successful public relations business.

Virginia Graham says she's "breathtakingly persistent and rationally determined. Energy can be dissipated but can then be reborn through knowledge to revitalize you."

Jockey Walter Blum is unbelievably determined. Can you imagine that this great jockey is allergic to animal hair and dust? He found it out in the early 1950s, just after he started riding professionally. He started wheezing and had a lot of trouble breathing. For a while it looked as if he would have to give up riding, but he was so determined to be a great jockey that he would do anything for his profession. He went to many doctors, and no one knew what the problem was. Finally he went to an allergist and was tested for everything until finally they found out about his allergy. He has to take many shots continually to stay on the tracks, but he says it's worth it to ride his beloved horses.

Now don't confuse will with persistence. You can will something and then rationalize and change your will. But the greater your imagination, the greater your determination. The more clearly you can see your goal in your mind's eye—the more you can image-in (imagine) to your mind what you want, the more determined and persistent you will be. Every person I talked to prefaced their enormous determination by saying if it's something they *really* want. It isn't a matter of just willing something —that's an empty mental process with not much to back it up—but getting a *clear* picture of what you really desire and hanging in there till it's yours.

Do you want to write a book? Start with one page a day or even half a page a day—and in a week you've got either seven or three-and-a-half pages—a beginning.

Imagine yourself sitting with an agent (first step to selling it) and having him or her represent you with a publisher. Imagine sitting with an editor in front of whom sits your manuscript. Imagine the thrill of seeing your book in a store window and then seeing people walk up and buy it. Now if you can get yourself fired up enough with these scenes of success, you will become more and more determined to start and finish your book. And if you finish it and get a few rejections, don't let that stop you—try to get the people who turned you down to tell you why they did. Then, if you agree with them that your book needs more action, or less action, make the changes, and keep on submitting, and eventually you'll get published. My first book was rejected by eight publishers before number nine took it, and it is doing very well in hard-cover and paperback.

There was an ad the other day in the *New York Times* about how a number one best seller was turned down countless times and went on to become a smashing success.

How the black sheep of the publishing industry became a #1 best seller. In the entire history of publishing, the dramatic success of *Winning through Intimidation* is without parallel. After being flatly rejected by major publishers, it is astonishing that the book even came to be printed.

How did this black sheep emerge from total rejection to the pinnacle of the publishing industry?

> Rumors abound—some almost legendary—regarding this unprecedented rags to riches achievement. Instead of being intimidated by the "experts"—who claimed there was no market for a book like this—the author kept in mind one of his most basic definitions: "An expert is merely a guy who knows all the reasons why you can't do something."

One well-known editor in chief in New York got fired not long ago because the last seven of her rejections went to other publishers and became best sellers. Always remember that a rejection—*any* rejection—is just one person's opinion. And what one person hates, another could love.

If you want to be a singer and feel you have some talent, go to showcases (places, usually bars, where amateurs perform), and sing. If you've got the guts to get up in front of an audience, half the battle is won. Or maybe you'd like to study singing. Find a good teacher, and begin. And if you don't like the first teacher, try another, or another, until you find someone with whom you have rapport. But don't give up. If you really truly want to sing, don't let anything or anybody stand in the way.

It may take a while to make money at what you'd really like to do, so do it before or after your paying job. If you're a secretary and want to write, you can write in the morning, at lunch, and at night. If you're a shoe salesman and want to sing, you can practice anytime, go to showcases at night, and audition for shows on your lunch break.

Just know what you really want, imagine what fun it will be when you're successful at it, and be persistent until you get it. Don't let anybody—including yourself— talk you out of it. And you won't, if your persistence is as strong as your desire.

III
Emotional Energy

7
LOVE
AND
THE WORLD
WILL LOVE
WITH YOU

Love is caring. Nothing more and nothing less. Most people try to give it a bigger or deeper meaning, but it all boils down to caring. Caring for yourself, caring for another, caring for lots of others. Being "in love" is more of a personal ego trip—caring for one terrific person exclusively who makes us feel that we're terrific (someone once said that love is recognizing our own consciousness in another).

What's caring? Caring means giving a damn about something—anything—from the war in Southeast Asia to war in general (that's loving peace)—from the New York

Mets to baseball in general—from the person you share your bed with to people in general. You can care for your little baby or children all over the world—care for your dog or all animals in general. Caring is love. Love is caring. One of the best ways to love a person is to make him or her feel important. This is the basis of all happiness—our self-image. This is the most important part of loving or caring for children. Making them feel important.

If a child feels he's excess baggage, that he's nothing, that his opinions mean nothing, that he's worth little, how can we expect him or her to try to accomplish something? How can we expect him or her to be able to give love when he feels so unworthy of it?

The terrible pain of being unloved is not the absence of love but seeing ourselves as being unlovable. And the only way of seeing ourselves as being lovable is by giving love and having it returned. And the place to start is to care for yourself. First get into the physical regime of the yeast and vites (you must admit I *am* persistent!) and get the bod in great shape. Then once you are relaxed and energy is flowing instead of being trapped in tension in your muscles, you will begin to have greater control over your emotions, and you will begin to become more positive. You will begin to like yourself, and that's the real beginning, the first step, to love.

One day shortly after I had submitted my manuscript to my publisher, I had a date with my good friend Kevin Sanders. Kevin and I met for the first time the first morning we co-hosted the "A.M. New York" show together on ABC. He's a darling, funny, warm, lovable, and whimsical man, but I had no idea how together he is until we started having breakfast after the show and we discussed everything from John Lilly's experiments with the porpoises to the philosophy of man's impersonal life.

Kevin was a little late and told me he had just left Warren Avis and a fascinating discussion. He had wanted to call me to join them but had left my phone number home. I asked who is Warren Avis, and he said the man who started Avis "We Try Harder" Rent-A-Car, and a brilliant researcher and author of man's emotional and cultural changes in society. He's written two books, *Shared Participation*, published by Doubleday, and *The Art of Sharing*, published by Simon & Schuster. Kevin then told me that Warren had done a thorough and exhaustive research with computers on what is love and had come out with a one-word answer. Because I had just written a whole chapter on love for my new book, I excitedly asked him what the one-word answer is and he said, "caring."

I could hardly believe my ears. I ran into my den and brought out my manuscript and showed him the opening line of my chapter on love—"Love is caring." I told Kevin I'd been contemplating love for a long time without all the subjective, emotional, romantic jazz that usually accompanies it, and I'd finally decided that "caring" was the word. But I told him I had to meet Warren Avis and find out how his computers came out with the same answer. I called Warren several times in Michigan where he has his American Behavioral Science Labs but was unable to reach him. They said he travels a great deal and would be back in a few days.

The next day my phone rang and it was Warren in New York. He knew about me from Kevin, and we met that afternoon. He explained about his striving to effect culture changes in society—that if we could change from conflict to problem solving and really work together, we could certainly be more successful and happier—that it would mean a better world for all of us. I was terribly impressed with Warren—he's a very dynamic man. And I couldn't wait to hear about the computer and his research on love, so I dove right in and asked how it all happened. He told me that he believes that the Western religions teaching that true love is selfless is an untruth, but that thinking it and proving it are two different things. He set about to prove it.

He hired Catholic priests and ministers from different churches. He worked with the Baptist seminary schools —in fact, today Warren is responsible for the Baptists' having changed their doctrine from selflessness to self-awareness. Anyway, he got a lot of religious teachers to work with him on the project. He said they used a wall as big as my whole apartment and nailed up all the philosophies and psychologies since recorded time. This took many months of research. Then they ran them through computers and came up with the answer—but it wasn't a one-word definition as Kevin had said, but three words. Love is "caring plus fulfillment."

I argued that if you truly care, *that's* your fulfillment.

In other words, if someone adopted ten homeless children, it wouldn't be a "selfless" deed because the action gave the person pleasure or he or she wouldn't have done it. Warren agreed but said he added fulfillment because a lot of people didn't understand about caring meaning fulfillment. Then he asked me if I have a brother or a sister. I said one of each. He said that I should imagine that my brother was drowning in a river and I was standing on the bank, unable to swim a stroke. If I dived in and drowned, everyone would say what a selfless thing I did, but that's not true. If I hadn't dived in—if I had just stood there and allowed him to drown—I wouldn't have been able to face my family or friends—or myself. I had to dive in, even though I knew I would drown. I would have done it for self-fulfillment, not selflessness (or self-moreness instead of selflessness).

What is caring? Caring is taking care of—taking care of the people and things around you. Watering your plants . . . remembering your husband's birthday . . . feeding the turtle . . . holding your wife's hand to let her know you're there taking care of her when she finds out her mother died . . . walking softly so as not to waken your roommate. When we care for someone or something, it makes us feel supergood. Caring gives us a meaning to life. When we care for ourselves (take care of ourselves) we are better people than when we treat ourselves badly or neglect ourselves.

And it's not possible to care for things and people outside ourselves if we don't start with ourselves. How can we give of our mentality if we haven't fed our minds with knowledge? If there's nothing there, there's nothing to give. The same with our bodies. If our bodies are tense and nervous (all negative), how can we impart lovingness to those around us? Just as there are carriers of typhoid and other diseases, there are carriers of nervous break-downs. How selfish to wish our negative emotions (jeal-ousy, hate, fear, etc.) on people, animals, and things around us. If you really care for someone, you'll want to make him or her happy. And happiness is giving love and not giving fear or anger or your own insecurity.

Jack Benny, the most loved of all comedians, gave so much of himself. And he was such a kind person—he never joked at another's expense, only his own. His humor was always poking fun at himself—he was a skinflint and an egomaniac, he said. And of course he was just the opposite, and everyone loved him because they felt better after being around him.

No one can live without love of somebody or some-thing, and the more love we are capable of giving, the more we will get back, and the happier and more fulfilled our lives will be.

Dr. Hutschnecker says we must make a distinction between love and being in love. "To be in love is a marvel-ous state of intoxication, like champagne that goes to your head. It's a peak sensation which unfortunately can-not be maintained. Love on the other hand is a deep emo-tion that originates from a need and matures into a deep feeling of relatedness, the desire to share with another human being feelings and experiences all one's life. Love is caring and always considering the feelings and needs of another. It's not a question of what do I get out of a relationship but a desire to give because of a will and a joy to give."

Ginger Rogers believes that God is love—her own personal love. Ginger is a beautiful woman and an unbelievable sixty-four years old. She looks more than thirty years younger, and the most incredible thing about her is her vitality. At an age when most people are taking life easy, she opened for the first time in her life in a nightclub act in New York at the Waldorf Astoria. She sings, she dances, and she's great. Surprisingly, Ginger is a real intellectual—a thinker at all times. She says that most people don't use nearly all their mental capacities. Her whole existence revolves around her relationship with God. She says all her energy and strength stem from her understanding and love of God, and the one book to which she attributes making the biggest change in her life is *Science and Health with a Key to the Scriptures* by Mary Baker Eddy. Ginger believes that God and good and love are interchangeable, and that this way of thinking has helped to make her the vital person she is.

Sammy Cahn wrote in a song, "Look to Your Heart" from the 1954 production of *Our Town*, "Speak your love to those who seek your love." But maybe we should speak our love to all those who touch our lives—and it will come back a thousandfold.

Howard Cosell's most important success in his opinion

is the success of his marriage for over thirty years. He believes that love is the most important element in the world
but that many people mistakenly think that sex is more
important. He says you can have a wild sex life and not
have love—.hat there are bigger things in life than sex—
that love transcends sex. People needing one another is the
most important thing. He says that a successful marriage
doesn't depend on sex after the marriage has established
itself. He says it is astounding, however, that the same
woman could stay in love with him for thirty-one years.
(He's only joking—he says he's a terrific husband!)

Mae West, that great superstar of all time, disagrees
with Howard, however. She says that sex is great, but it
can never be as great as when you're in love—that sex can
then drive you mad.

I believe the truth of the matter lies between the two.
Sex without love is not as great as with love, and love
without sex is missing an important part. Sex is the closest
two people can get physically, and if you are also close
emotionally, you're an unbeatable team. But it's not enough
just to love someone—you've got to express your love and
make the one you care for *feel* loved.

I've already quoted Ralph Waldo Emerson, my all-time
favorite philosopher, but he's so great I want to now quote
him on love:

> The private and tender relation of one to one is the
> enchantment of human life; which, like a certain
> divine rage and enthusiasm, seizes one man at one

period, and works a revolution in his mind and body; unites him to his race, pledges him to the domestic and civic relations, carries him with new sympathy into nature, enhances the power of the senses, opens the imagination, adds to his character heroic and sacred attributes, establishes marriage, and gives permanence to human society . . . he touched the secret of the matter, who said of love, "All other pleasures are not worth its pains."

In love, trust is very important. David Viscott, M.D., says in his book, *How to Live with Another Person*, "Trust is the creation of two people who care for each other and believe in the relationship between them."

And Dr. Eugene Scheimann says in *Sex Can Save Your Heart and Life* that love is a man's and a woman's first and single most important need from the first breath of life to the last.

Can a person have energy without love? I don't believe a person can exist without love. Years ago an experiment was made in two foundling homes. In one, the nurses were instructed not to touch or talk to any of the babies. In the second, the nurses were told to pick up the babies as often as possible and to fondle them and talk to them. At the end of a year, every baby had died at the first orphanage, and all the babies were healthy and thriving at the second one.

Dr. Mary Ann Bartusis, a member of the Committee on Women and the American Psychiatric Association, says:

Love is important to your life—so important that you can die without it. It has been proven that children and very small infants can die if denied love. Without love, an adult can become so depressed that he or she may commit suicide.

We are human and need love, affection, and attention, and when we don't get it we become morose, depressed, and physically sick. Don't ever forget that the body and mind and emotions function as one unit. If one part is sick it must affect the other parts. If your emotional life is empty—if no one cares for you and you care for no one —it will totally affect your life. Either it will create body tension (trapped energy) or a physical depression (no energy). When you're tense you get in your own way, and any energy is used up in muscular tension. When you're depressed, you don't give a fig what happens, and a lethargy permeates your body and drains you of all energy.

So without love, or caring, for someone or something, desire will be missing—desire for *anything*—and with the lack of desire, there's a lack of energy.

But when you love, or care, for someone or something, desire will take over—desire to please, desire to do, desire to take care of—and this desire will energize your whole being. Just remember back to when you fell in love—or better yet, fall in love again (you can even do this with your present mate, if necessary), and you'll see what I mean. Your imagination will be loosed, and you'll have energy enough to conquer the world—or at least your lover!

8
IT'S NOT A NERVOUS BREAKDOWN— IT'S AN EGO BREAKDOWN

Everybody talks about nervous breakdowns, which sounds okay if you say it fast. But it implies that the whole nervous system falls apart—just breaks down and stops working. Now this just isn't so. At our very worst, in the middle of the worst trauma that could hit us and as upset as we can get, our nervous systems are still functioning. We can still walk around. We're still able to drink a glass of water and answer intelligent questions. We may not *want* to do these things, but we're able to. The wanting is the key.

When something happens that lowers our self-esteem or almost destroys it completely, we stop *wanting* to do things. It's a chore to answer the phone, or eat, or do anything, because we feel so nothing that nothing is what we want to do.

"If she stopped loving me, I must be unlovable. I must be a creep who isn't worth anyone caring for. No one will ever love me again because I'm such a nothing."

"If my boss fired me after I tried so hard to do a good job, I must be a real jerk. I mean, if I were any good, if I had talent, he wouldn't have fired me. I must be a worthless person. Only worthless people get treated this way."

Now, lots of people get blows to their egos every day, and they don't fall apart. Well, just like there are thousands of different personal chemical balances (we don't all get the flu in a flu epidemic), and millions of different fingerprints, everyone's ego is different. Some of us have strong egos, able to withstand insults, slights, or traumas, and others of us have weak egos that crumble at the slightest affront. Our mothers and fathers, teachers and friends helped us form our ego structures when we were kids, and most of us carry their opinions of us through life. And it's *only* their opinion. The pity of it is we start to believe them, and it becomes *our* opinion of ourselves.

Maybe we were shy as kids, and dad, who always wanted a football player who would carry on in his business of making steel ball bearings (a real "man's job"), resented our quiet, artistic ways, and his opinion was we weren't quite okay.

Maybe we were tomboyish and mom always wanted a "little lady" who baked cookies and loved to clean the house, and all we wanted was to play baseball with the guys on the block (and we were a better player than any guy and this made mom even sadder). Anyway, mom made us feel inferior as a woman (girls don't *do* that sort of thing) and we grew up with a weak and battered ego. Well just as it was only their opinion then, it's only our opinion now, and we can change that opinion. Barbara Walters, George McGovern, and Barbra Streisand changed their opinions of themselves and strengthened their egos at the same time, just as each one of us can do so it will be impossible to have an ego breakdown.

The three of them, Barbara, George, and Barbra, started out doubting themselves but set out to prove the self-doubt wrong. Barbara Walters used intellectual achievement at school as a refuge from the loneliness caused by going to five different schools before she was fifteen and not knowing a soul in each one, so high grades became her ego buffer, and as she got into writing, she became more successful, and her ego strength grew with her success.

George McGovern concentrated on public speaking in school and developed a wonderful style of combining honesty and candor with a forceful manner of getting his ideas across. He seems to be a humble man (can a politician really be humble?) but political success has made his ego much stronger than it was in school.

Barbra Streisand started childhood with a very weak,

insecure ego, but through determination she developed her unique singing style (it took years and years of practice singing in front of the mirror); she's now one of the few superstars, and her ego grew with her.

Dr. Arnold Hutschnecker says there's great confusion about ego. "Ego does not mean to throw one's weight around. Psychoanalytically, ego is the expression of the Self striving for self-fulfillment. Ego is to do the best one can do for oneself before one can do for others."

Most of us are embarrassed by our egos. When we pass a mirror or our reflection in a window we sneak a glance and guiltily wonder if anyone saw us. Why should we feel guilty about wanting to look good? There's so much guilt around that this is only a teensy one, but I believe it colors everything we do. If we can't feel proud of our looks and happy to see a well-cared-for body or a nice new hairstyle, then we're being dumb and illogical.

I think it started with the Pilgrims, who taught that anything fun was bad and for God's sake don't appear too attractive. I enjoy looking at good-looking, well-cared-for people, and it makes my stomach turn to see a huge gut hanging over a low-slung pair of pants, or a ton of arm blubber hanging from a short-sleeved summer dress. It's not only ugly and distasteful looking, it's downright suicidal. Carrying fifty extra pounds puts an enormous strain on a body, particularly the heart. Just imagine carrying around a fifty-pound suitcase every minute of the day, day in and day out. I'm rather tall and very healthy, and I can hardly lift a fifty-pound suitcase, much less carry it around all day. With all my energy, I would be depleted all too soon. I mean, you can only do so much of certain things—you only want to climb five flights of stairs once, you don't want to do it ten times an hour. Of course if you had to, you'd develop the leg muscles and eventually it would seem easy. But carrying extra pounds of blubber just doesn't make sense, and the person carrying it is so unhealthy that the fifty pounds never becomes easy, and the heart gets strained more and more every day till it just conks out.

A few years ago, before I got into yeast and vites, I used to get depressed between anxiety attacks, so I decided to see a psychiatrist—or psychologist, I forget which. Anyway, he was very nice and I worked with him several times. On about my third visit he told me I had the weakest ego he'd ever encountered (my brother still doesn't believe this story and tells everybody about my weak little ego). The doctor said with all I had going for me—youth, a career as an actress, many boyfriends and girl friends, a beautiful apartment in Beverly Hills (this was before I fell in love with New York)—I should have had the world on a string. But I didn't. I was getting in my own way. Not until I cut out all the sugar and junk foods and cigarettes and built my body up and got rid of all the anxiety and depression and had the tension turned into active energy did I fully appreciate what the doctor had said.

To have a really healthy and strong ego you must concentrate on accomplishing what you consider important until you build up a healthy sense of self-worth. When I got rid of the tension and really became a doer, my ego got stronger because I was beginning to do some things that I felt were important. And the more I accomplished, the stronger my sense of self-worth, or my ego, became.

All the people with whom I discussed this agreed that the older they became the better their self-image became. Everyone I interviewed, without exception, said that as they worked and accomplished, their egos grew stronger and more healthy in proportion to their accomplishments.

David Susskind says his ego is much stronger and healthier now than when he was a kid. He recognized the need for accomplishment when he was very young and very unsure of himself, he decided that he should win academic distinction in high school, and he did. He won scholarships in school. As he's grown older he's gotten much more successful. He is now recognized as a producer of merit, and he no longer feels he's got to prove himself. Because of this not only did his ego get stronger, but he's gotten more tolerance for the human race, and for himself.

Arlene Dahl had a tremendous inferiority because of her beautiful mother. She lived in her own little shell until the age of eighteen, when she discovered mascara (until then she swears you couldn't see her eyes, her lashes and brows were so pale—and she felt like a complete nothing).

Jim Bouton was always a pretty confident kid because his family was very supportive of his self-esteem. "I got lots of love at home which gave me a secure feeling to be an individual. They gave me lots of praise. However, my ego is stronger now because my tangible success is on a larger scale than when I was a kid."

Virginia Graham had a weak ego throughout her childhood, and not until she was thirty-eight did she find herself; her ego was nourished through her television work. When "Girl Talk" first went on the air she was fairly confident it would be a success because she truly likes people and likes to communicate with them, but when the show became such a big hit and ran for so many years (and would probably still be running had she and the network not had a falling-out over contracts), her ego became much stronger than it had ever been in her life. When people recognize you on the street and stop you to chat because they feel they know you and instinctively like you, as happened to Virginia constantly, it's bound to have a good effect and make your self-image grow.

Jackie Mason believes that most entertainers have sick egos. I disagree with him. Of course, some entertainers do —but so do some plumbers, morticians, and manicurists. Because a person has a desire to find love and approbation through applause is no sign of sickness. It's not self-destructive or other-destructive. Sickness, in my opinion, is when you hurt yourself or put yourself down—or deliberately hurt another through hostility, criticism, or any other negative not meant to make yourself or another person happy.

Sammy Cahn, the prolific songwriter (he's written lyrics to over fifty top songs, four of which won the Oscar:

"Three Coins in the Fountain," "Call Me Irresponsible," "High Hopes," and "All the Way"; and others just as great like "My Kind of Town," "The Second Time Around," "Be My Love," "It's Magic," "Bei Mir Bist Du Schoen," etc., etc., etc.) has an enormous ego that his success helped to build from a not-so-confident childhood—possibly because of being the only boy with four sisters. But everybody finds him adorable and his ego refreshing. He's not hurting anybody. In fact, he's a very entertaining person. He's the first songwriter in history who went on the ultimate ego trip—he starred on Broadway in a show all about himself, *Words and Music,* and he was so terrific that it played for months and then went to London, where it was also a big hit. Sammy's "on" all the time, but his ego's not offensive because he's so entertaining and fun.

Mohammed Ali is another nonentertainer with a gigantic ego that is entertaining. Mohammed is *all* ego, but he performs and I love it. He appears to be all wrapped up in himself, but he's not. He's a colorful guy who makes life more exciting, but he started out as a scared little black kid in Louisville, and it wasn't until he started winning fights that his ego began to grow.

Bobby Riggs has a big ego, which tennis strengthened from his earlier shaky self-confidence, but a big sense of humor goes along with it. Before Billie Jean King clobbered him on the courts, he was tooting his horn about being a male chauvinist pig and how Billie Jean didn't stand a chance. He and the much-touted event were fun.

Back to show-biz entertainers—Al Jolson, with his

"you ain't seen nuthin' yet" billed himself as the World's Greatest Entertainer, and addressed himself in the third person ("Jolie wants to take a walk"). He had an ego you could fly to Mars on, but people loved it.

And Ethel Merman's cockiness is deserved—she's great! Let's face it, if she didn't think she were terrific, do you think she'd have the chutzpah to stand on stage (I should say *conquer* the stage, 'cause that's what she does) and belt out the way she does?

Monique Van Vooren, the gorgeous blonde Belgian entertainer—she sings and dances, as well as acts—says she has a strong ego. She says it's too strong to be healthy, and she feels this was caused by a lack of response and support from her family when she was a child. She always wanted to be something, so her ego grew with her desire. Her family made her feel in the way. Her mother wanted a boy, and her father ignored her altogether. When you look at this beautiful woman, it's hard to imagine a deprived childhood, and Monique has worked hard to overcome this.

Buddy Rich is acclaimed as the world's greatest drummer. He's been at it since he was a little kid. He started out as a tap dancer and was one of the best child tappers around in vaudeville. Then he changed from tapping to rapping and became a kid drummer known as Baby Traps. He says he has a super-healthy superego, and it's strictly because of his talent. He knows he's a great drummer, and he works hard at staying great because he feels that without his sticks he's nothing.

Howard Cosell says his ego is strong in some areas—it s strong in what he does, his work. He started out in life with tremendous insecurity for several reasons. First, his parents never had money (which made him decide early that money was important to him), and he grew up Jewish in the age of Adolph Hitler, which psychologically made him very insecure. He decided to become an honor student in high school, and from that time on he was always at the top of every class. Achievement made his ego stronger and healthier. Then he went to law school and edited the law review and ultimately became Phi Beta Kappa. He practiced law for a while and then decided to go into the fields of sports and communications. He says he never would have changed jobs if he hadn't had enormous confidence brought about by earlier successes.

Sheila MacRae says she has a very strong and healthy ego brought about by a sense of accomplishment in her early years. Her parents and her teachers were all extremely supportive of her endeavors, and they gave her a strong sense of self-worth.

Alexander Cohen says he's astounded by his importance. But lots of times when he's recognized on the street and people wave at him, he's brought down drastically when they shout, "Hello, Earl!" He looks amazingly like Earl Wilson, the columnist, and lots of people make the mistake. (Earl is a pussycat, one of the darlingest of all people, and I'll have to ask him if people say to him "Hello Alex!") Alex says he knew from the age of four that he wanted to be a theatrical producer, and from that age on he was confident that he would be successful—in fact he thought of nothing else. Maybe it's coincidental, but his father died when Alex was four, and his mother was too preoccupied with her life to pay much attention to Alex, so maybe that's why he escaped into the dream world of entertainment.

Henny Youngman says that as a little kid people were always trying to put him down, but he wouldn't let them. He was a show-off as a kid and always wanted to be a comic. His ego grew with his comic success. He says he's always been ahead of his time—he thought of Dial-A-Joke and sold it to the phone company and got an enormous amount of publicity for himself because of it. His success on "Laugh In" brought him national attention (where before he was known mostly to Easterners, particularly New Yorkers), and this helped his ego a lot.

Hildegarde worked very hard for her talent, and this talent is what gives her ego-support. She is one of the most disciplined and hard-working women in show business, constantly rehearsing to improve her act, but this is why she believes in herself.

Walter Blum is one of the most famous jockeys in the world, and in 1973 he became the sixth rider in North America ever to ride 4,000 winners, ranking behind Willie Shoemaker, Johnny Longden, Eddie Arcaro, Steve Brooks, and William Hartack. He's very shy and self-effacing and says that the only thing that gives him confidence is that he knows that he's a great rider. In 1969 he was elected president of the Jockeys' Guild and has held that post ever since, and the fact that all the other jockeys like and admire him as much as they do also gave his ego a big boost.

When my first book came out in 1973 and I was making a lot of television appearances, I went to Washington, D.C., to go on the "Panorama" show. The one-hour show had only two guests: Dr. Neil Solomon, the secretary of health and mental hygiene of the state of Maryland and author of *The Truth about Weight Control*, and myself. I was told by the producer of the show that they were looking for some fireworks and they felt that Dr. Solomon, being a well-known doctor and not too hip on vitamins, would take me on and not demolish me too greatly—but they also knew that I'm a fighter for what I believe in, and I also know my business about nutrition. On the plane ride down I skimmed through the doctor's book and made a lot of mental notes.

Well, the time came, the lights went on, and away we went. At the beginning Dr. Solomon was quite nasty to me and very anti-everything I would say about nutrition. He made fun of my lack of formal education in nutrition and implied that I knew nothing—that no one but a doctor could possibly know anything about *anything.* He got angrier and angrier on the show, and the producer and director got happier and happier. They felt a donnybrook was a'comin'. But I had taken my yeast milkshake that morning (why should that morning have been different from all the rest?) and I was really enjoying myself. I felt his anger was totally unjustified, and the madder he got, the cooler I stayed.

About midway through the show he was putting me down unmercifully and saying that he had all the credentials and I had none. I pointed out that doctors are trained in healing the sick, but they have a paucity of training about how to keep you well; in fact, only a small percentage of all the medical schools in the United States have even a one-week course in nutrition, so how can anyone get any information on vitamins or nutrition from doctors? (This was after he stated that no one should take a vitamin without first checking with his or her doctor.) He really blew his cool. Fortunately a commercial break was slated, and we broke for a few minutes. During this time I tried to show him that he couldn't get me angry and that his anger was only turning the audience off him, because if I were such a nothing, why was he debating with me on TV and why would he get angry with me, why not just dismiss me as a dodo?

Well, when we went back on the air, his whole attitude changed, and we started rationally discussing everything from the vitamin A in beef liver to pantothenic acid. After the show he apologized to me for having been so vitriolic during the first half. I asked him why he had been so mean to me, and he said he had thought I was some dumb dame who knew nothing—a real phony—and wanted to unmask me on the air. Then I asked him what changed his attitude, and he said that after a while he could see that I was sincere and that I really believed in what I was talking about. He said that even though he didn't agree with everything I believed in, he had newfound respect for me.

I certainly felt better after that, but my confidence zoomed two days later when I received an official-looking letter, opened it, and on the official state of Maryland stationery with the governor's seal and all was a message from Neil (we parted on a first-name basis). He wanted me to serve as a member of the advisory board of the Department of Health and Mental Hygiene of the state of Maryland for a public health-service program to be presented over WBAL-TV, the NBC affiliate in Baltimore. Within a few weeks he arranged several guest spots for me on TV shows where he was appearing, and I found out what a terrific person he is (and he has gotten much more into nutrition and vitamins now). Before this I felt secure in my knowledge of nutrition, but this really boosted my self-worth and made me feel terrific. When other people back up your own feelings of worthiness, it's a real ego booster; isn't that what audiences do for an entertainer, and isn't that why we all, or most of us, try to please other people?

The only time ego is obnoxious is when there's no sense of humor along with it, and the only time ego is ridiculous is when there's no talent or performance to back it up; but even then it can be funny—if you have a sense of humor!

Johnny Carson, one of the world's funniest people, expresses his ego by taking on a challenge, proving he can master it, and then walking away from it. He mastered archery, golf, astronomy, and many other subjects. As a kid he became the Great Carsoni after he learned how to do lots of difficult magic tricks, which talent lifted him and his shaky ego way above his schoolmates and made him feel important. He has proved to himself that there's nothing so far that he wants to do that he can't do, and that's very ego-satisfying.

The word "ego" is from the Latin and means "I." When you assert your self or "I" and write a poem or make a movie or bake a cake, it's a natural expression. Animals can't do it. Animals have no ego, no idea of self—and animals can't create anything except other animals.

Everybody in the whole world needs ego-support. Why do people get married or live together? A person finds someone who feels he's the greatest—who loves him better than anyone else in the world and makes him feel important—and he marries that person so he'll have someone to build up his ego.

We all need someone or something to feel important because we all feel unimportant on our own. It started at birth when we were the center of mummy and daddy's world and then slowly we realized that we weren't; we were on our own, and that's tough to handle. Everybody needs to feel loved and needed. Everybody without exception.

Thomas Edison, Abraham Lincoln, Maria Callas, Irving Berlin, Gloria Steinem, Jonas Salk, Christiaan Barnard, Peggy Lee, Earl Wilson, Steve Allen, Bella Abzug—all these people were or are driven to create. And the people who aren't creative are driven to sex, and affairs, and multiple marriages, and the people whose egos are stifled are unhappy and miserable.

How dull life would be if we didn't have egos. We'd have no books, no music, no buildings, no paintings, no films—no nuthin'! And most importantly, nuthin' would be any fun if we couldn't show off just a little bit. When you accomplish something—anything—worthwhile, you begin to respect yourself, and then others do, and this is the first step to liking yourself (see next chapter). I believe this is the bottom line of happiness—that from which all happiness springs, and without which you can have no happiness.

9
HOW TO FALL
IN LIKE
WITH
YOURSELF

One principle, philosophy, outlook, emotion, or whatever you feel like calling it, will make every other thing in your life fall in place. It's the thing that can make your life fun and exciting, and can make all your far-outest dreams come true—dreams of success, love, health, friends, etc. It's the most tremendous thing you can learn, because without it nothing is possible.

You must like yourself. Not stand in front of a mirror and gaze longingly like a nut. Not selfishly think only of yourself. These aren't expressions of liking yourself, these are neurotic ways of trying to convince yourself that the self-loathing that you feel inside is wrong. "I don't hate myself . . . see how I go out and buy myself all these super clothes . . . I don't really hate myself . . ."

You must like yourself. I mean really care for yourself, deeply feel a warm sense of self-worth, get rid of all guilt for wanting the best for yourself. Then and only then can you really begin to like other people. Everything starts with liking yourself. Now you might say, "How stupid— of course I like myself." But do you really? Or are you usually putting yourself down for having a lousy memory ("I can't remember a thing"), being unlucky ("I'm the unluckiest person in the world"), and on and on with other downers about yourself? Sure it may be hard to remember things, but your memory is like a muscle; the more you use it the stronger it gets. An actor has a good memory because he uses it a lot to memorize scripts. You don't get mad at yourself for being a lousy quarterback or a terrible operatic soprano, because you never play football or sing opera and would hardly compare yourself to Joe Namath or Maria Callas. If you feel your memory could be improved, improve it. And if you truly like yourself, you will. And if you don't like yourself you'll go on forever complaining about how you can't remember a thing. My point is, give yourself a break. Don't down yourself. If there's something you can do to improve yourself—and who can't???—then do it.

Most of us have been programmed since childhood to doubt ourselves. Isn't it a pity most parents don't realize they really do shape a child's future by the actions and reactions the child observes? If the child senses the parent has no confidence in himself or in the child, he'll also have no confidence in himself. We get messed up 'cause the people around us are messed up when we're little kids.

People will accept us at our own evaluation. If you like yourself and think you're terrific, most people around you will too.

If you don't like yourself, don't despair. There's a foolproof, 100 percent effective way of changing this around. Let's assume that all your life you never were too crazy about yourself. You realize the importance of self-image and how powerful a good self-image can be, and you've tried to tell yourself you're really a nice person— not a knockout, but really nice. You've tried to sell yourself this, but it doesn't work. You just won't or can't buy it. You really don't believe you're an okay person. How can you convince yourself you're really worthwhile? There is something positive you can do to make yourself like yourself. It's an easy, active exercise and it's *guaranteed* to work.

Before I give it to you, let me tell you of an experience I had when I started acting. I had just read Stanislavsky's *An Actor Prepares*, which is a fantastic book and tells all about how an actor readies himself from within for a part. There are lots of examples of how actors prepare emotionally for a particular part. Then I joined several acting groups with Clint Eastwood, Carolyn Jones, Richard Boone, James Whitmore, and a few other good actors, and one of the teachers, a well-known Broadway and Hollywood actor, showed his students how to pretend to be a tree or a dog, or any object. It was all mental and emotional. "Think like a tree and you will become one," he kept intoning. Well, I thought and thought and felt and felt, but I didn't become a tree. Oh, I guess I did a little bit. My arms felt a *little* bit like a tree as I held them patiently out, and they moved ever so slightly in the breeze. But I wasn't *totally* a tree. Something was missing.

Lucky for me someone gave me Michael Chekhov's book *To the Actor*. Chekhov took the completely opposite view. He stated that you don't start on the inside and work out with your thoughts, but on the outside, with your body, and work in. He showed that warmth and love are open, and fear and hate are closed. He gave physical exercises to open up—standing with your arms and legs spread open—and exercises to close up—sitting, hugging your knees in a semifetal position. There were many other exercises, and they all worked. If I were to imagine myself to be a tree, first I would do his opening exercise and feel really open like a tree and open to all the elements. And if I were to imagine myself to be a boulder, I did his closing-up exercise and I would feel completely closed like a rock. Then when I played a part of a whimsical, fun-loving, warm, and funny girl, I knew the feeling of openness; and when I played a part of a cynical, fearful, angry girl, I knew how to close up.

I decided to test out the exercises to see if they really worked or were just my imagination. After practicing my exercises for about a week, I had a friend of mine sit on

154

my couch and I stood with my back to him. Without moving a muscle, I mentally and emotionally opened up and closed up and he "felt" every one I did. He guessed twenty-five out of twenty-five, so I proved to myself that it works. Up until this time I had thought *everything* started in the mind. When I got anxious or depressed, I thought I could will myself out of these feelings—this was before I discovered nutritional yeast, chapter 1! With Chekhov's exercises I began to see that the mind, emotions, and body are one, and that the mind cannot be in control if the body is badly treated and out of shape—a mess. And of course the body won't be in shape if the mind doesn't care enough to put it in shape.

There is positively something you can do to make yourself like yourself. You can't will it to happen. You can't just say, "I'm going to start liking myself better," because it won't work. You have to *do* something to *make* liking yourself seem logical—everything in this book is logical because *I'm* logical. You have to do something so that your self will say, "Hey, I'm a pretty terrific person—I accomplished something." You can start with something small, such as promising yourself that every day for a week you'll climb the three flights of stairs to your apartment instead of taking the elevator. It sounds simple, and it is simple. There's just one catch. Once you promise yourself something you *must* keep the promise, or you'll really hate yourself for not keeping it. That's why you start out with something simple and fairly easy to do. Like, "I'll wait till 10:00 A.M. for my first cigarette."

Of course, it's a good idea to make the accomplishment something that's good for your health (climbing stairs, stopping smoking) or otherwise beneficial to you. Maybe promise yourself to learn how to play the guitar and practice ten minutes a day. Or start taking my morning milkshake for one month. Set a time limit; you can always extend it if you want. But your mind's gotta have a limit to work toward. It can't be forever—that's too much to expect from yourself. But a week, two weeks, a month—that's terrific. You can try only one martini before dinner for a week instead of two; it's only for a week, and what a super feeling of self-reliance comes over you when you see that you *can* rely on your self when you ask yourself to do something.

Marlene Dietrich is a very disciplined person. Once, when she was very young, she made herself go out in freezing weather without a coat just to prove to herself she could do it. Her mental discipline is fantastic, and it pushed her right to the top. Now what you ask yourself to do can be progressively harder after each accomplishment. You can make a game out of it and keep coming up with things to make yourself do. It's fun to find little things and do them and feel better after doing them—you might be surprised at how good you'll feel afterwards.

But remember—once you make the commitment to yourself to do something, you MUST carry through. If not, the reverse will happen and you will *despise* yourself for not doing it. That's the reason for the short period of time—to make it not too difficult to do, and to insure success with just a little discipline and determination.

Now after doing things for yourself, you can try doing little worthwhile things for other people. Once you give yourself any job to do and you do it, you'll feel great. You don't have to start with big-time-save-the-world kind of things, just little things that you'll accept as being good or kind or helpful to others. How's about holding a swinging door open after you've walked through so it doesn't slam into someone as it closes? Or getting up on a bus or subway and giving someone your seat, just out of kindness? Or sending someone a cute little friendship card just because you like him or her? You can tell someone how well he or she looks, what a terrific tie or hairdo —doing little things to make others feel important. In no time at all you'll begin to see and feel what a terrific person you are to do these little things for others.

Even when someone is nasty or curt, try to imagine that he or she is going through a terrible tragedy. His mother may be dying of cancer . . . she may have just found out she can never have children . . . his boss may have just given him a pink slip and he's got mortgage payments up to his ears . . . he may have just found out his wife's in love with another man . . . she may have just found out her husband's in love with another man. We always tend to think our problems are the biggest and the rest of the world has few troubles, but that ain't so; everyone has problems of some sort—boy, do we! Now, some of us have trained ourselves to try and mentally rise above them, but they still exist. No one is without troubles of some sort. And when you really become aware of this, it's easier to understand when people yell or are rude. You may not agree with what they're doing, but at least it softens the rudeness a little to have pity for the possibility of a tragedy in the yeller's life. A well-adjusted person who has a sense of self-worth doesn't have to be rude. In fact, if you like yourself, you'll like other people; and if you don't like yourself, you won't really like anybody.

The most important thing in life to us is our own self-importance. How important are we? What are we worth to ourselves and to others? If we can make ourselves feel important, we shall know happiness. And if we can make others feel important, we can make them happy—and ourselves, too. Take a nasty, surly person. You can be nice and smile at him—nothing. You can say, "Good morning"—and silence greets you. But make that person feel important, even in small ways, and he'll be happy—if only momentarily. We're here on earth—why, we ask. If we feel it's for nothing, how can we be happy? But if we feel it's for a reason, whatever the reason, we can feel worthwhile. And whatever we do to feel worthwhile, be it discovering uranium, visiting hospitals, becoming president, or whatever, is a logical and intelligent thing to do.

Tony Curtis, when he was Bernie Schwartz, used to hang around Sardi's in New York, and he wasn't too thrilled with himself. His self-image was Bronx deze, dem, and doze. If you see any of his early flicks you'll see that that image was hard for him to shake. But as soon as the studio changed his name to Jimmy Curtis he liked himself a little better; and then, when he changed it to Tony Curtis, his whole self-image changed. I mean, a Tony Curtis meant class, but a Bernie Schwartz, echhh! So if you don't like something about yourself, change it.

Most people don't like themselves because they don't know themselves. They don't know how terrific they can be. How they can really rely on themselves more than they can rely on anyone else in the world. After all, you're the only one you can control. You can't really control your husband or wife, children or friends, but you *can* control yourself. You can make yourself do anything you want. Just give yourself the command and follow through. What a way to get things accomplished.

Lucille Ball, that energetic redhead, answered a recent interviewer who asked her how she accounted for all the years of her TV success, "Very simply—I like myself." This is the same Lucille Ball whose high school drama coach said about her that she was "too shy and too reticent" to be an actress. She then flunked out of John Murray Anderson's drama school in New York, where she was told, "Try another profession, any other." Then she got pneumonia with complications that disabled her for three years. Besides physical pain, she lived through much emotional pain during her marriage to Desi Arnaz. She didn't start out liking herself—it took a lot of mental discipline—but what a payoff!

Lucille Ball set goals for herself and made herself do them. She was "too shy and too reticent" to be an actress—that was somebody else's opinion, not hers. She forced herself to perform in front of audiences to overcome her shyness She was told to "try another profession, any other"—well, she wanted to be an actress and she didn't care if she failed an acting course; she was going to be an actress. She set her goals, no matter how difficult, and forced herself to do them.

We can all do this. It's not difficult if we start out with simple things and build up to more difficult things. And no matter who we are, if we accomplish something we give ourselves to do we have to feel proud of ourselves; it just doesn't work any other way. This is one of the laws of the universe, and it is a law. It works every time, without exception.

You've been reading about all the pluses that happen when you begin to like yourself, but what about what happens when you don't like yourself? One thing for sure; you gotta resent other people because you will not be self-reliant, you'll be other-people-reliant, and we all know how little we can rely on most other people. You'll probably be disappointed a lot when people let you down, and of course this will lead to anger. You'll be mad a lot of the time at a lot of people. And jealous—oh, yeah—if you don't like yourself you'll think everybody around you is better than you, and you'll be envious of their looks, personalities, sex-appeal, or accomplishments. If you don't like yourself you'll tend to think most people don't like you—if I don't like me, why should they?—and you'll consciously or unconsciously be rude and selfish a lot of the time. You'll usually be unsure of yourself because of your inferiority feelings and think everyone else is superior.

You won't have much faith in yourself, and you'll be fearful of a lot of things. Actually all negative emotions are based on fear. Do you have any idea how draining fear is on our energy? Not to mention anger, jealousy, resentment, and all the other negatives you'll be filled with. And energy is what this book is all about.

I asked people I interviewed if they liked themselves and what they liked most and what, if anything, they disliked about themselves. I got some interesting answers. Virginia Graham likes best her honesty with herself; she says she talks aloud to herself a lot—which I do, too. She also likes her sense of humor, her ability to laugh, which gives her the strength to cope. Much pain in her earlier years built up a tremendous inner strength. Virginia had cancer in her thirties and the doctors said it was incurable, but her inner faith pulled her through the operation to a total cure. She had many personal tragedies in her life, but her incredible sense of humor—she's one of the funniest persons I've ever met—gave her a marvelous perspective, and she overcame every problem. The only thing Virginia doesn't like about herself is that she sticks by bad judgment. She also doesn't like the sound of silence, so she has a radio going constantly. But she says that's not as bad as the judgment thing, because fear keeps her from changing her judgment, and the radio thing is just loneliness.

Howard Cosell likes his moral courage the best—the fact that he stands for something. He's not afraid to take a stand on anything in which he believes.

Buddy Rich says he likes his ability to do something that's important and an accomplishment. He says he's not really thrilled with himself but with his talent.

George Barrie, the president of Fabergé and a very creative tycoon in the business world, likes his creative drive the best. He says creativity is the most important thing in his life, and he has taken Fabergé into producing motion pictures. He also hired Sammy Cahn to work for him, and they have co-written several songs. The only thing he dislikes about himself is any lack of creativity.

Serge Obolensky says he's an individualist who likes harmony around himself—he's a Libra and all Librans need harmony—and the thing he likes best about himself is his easy gregariousness; he really likes people. The thing he dislikes most is his temper.

Sammy Cahn likes his honesty with himself the best —he admits all his faults and sincerely tries to correct them. He says he dislikes his cunning.

Dr. Benjamin Frank likes his truthfulness the best but dislikes his impracticality.

Sheila MacRae says she gets along with everybody—I can attest to this—and tries to understand people. She never judges others. This is so important to personal freedom. "Judge not that you be not judged" is telling us that if we don't judge other people we also won't judge ourselves, and judging ourselves makes us hyper-critical and self-conscious and keeps us from acting freely and without undue caution.

Dr. Joyce Brothers likes the fact that she's now at the point where she does what she thinks is right instead of what other people think. She says this comes with emotional maturity.

Hildegarde likes her compassion for people the best and dislikes her impatience and resentfulness.

Arlene Dahl likes her attitude to life and other people, which is positive and has always been positive. She dislikes being late to appointments and says she's working hard on overcoming this.

Jim Bouton likes his concentration best, his candidness second best, and his sense of humor third best. He says his sense of humor has enabled him to get by situations that would have been awful had he not made them funny. He tells of a Christmas when he was a little kid and the family didn't have much money. He had some Christmas money for presents, but he lost it and was heartbroken. He didn't know what to do and was imagining waking up Christmas morning with hardly anything under the tree. Then he got a brainstorm. He went around the house and collected things like Bon Ami, bath soap, ashtrays (which he cleaned), Campbell's Pork and Beans, old socks, toothpaste tubes, old magazines, etc., etc., etc., and wrapped them all up in Christmas paper with bright ribbons and put them all under the tree. The family on

Christmas morning thought this was hilarious and had a wonderful Christmas, saved by Jim's fey sense of humor. Jim dislikes his temper the most.

David Susskind likes his honesty, givingness, receptivity, and sense of humor—he's got a great sense of humor. He says he believes he's a good person. He dislikes his striving for perfection and his demands on himself and other people.

Percy Sutton likes his compassion for people, honesty, and sense of humor the best; he's also a very funny man.

Henny Youngman says "I'm crazy about myself. I have a lot of laughs and I enjoy life and like to help people. I dislike the fact that I can't control my desire for food now, but I'm working on it."

It doesn't take a genius to see how important liking ourselves is—how it affects every second of our lives. And knowing that we can change our opinion of ourselves gives us enormous hope for happiness. Everyone I interviewed who told me of things they disliked about themselves also said they were working on changing these things, and they all said they had already changed a lot of things they didn't like about themselves through working on them. We don't have to accept a low opinion of ourselves which leads to self-dislike. We can start to slowly build a different self-image. You'll be amazed at how fast you'll begin to like yourself. This doesn't take weeks or years; it can start immediately.

But of course thinking about it doesn't cut it; you gotta do it. Go ahead, pick out some little thing that'll improve you in some way, no matter how small, and do it and see for yourself. See if you don't start feeling a little more self-reliant and start liking yourself a little more—which, if you keep it up, will be a lot more. What a super feeling; "Hey, I asked myself to do it and I *did* it. Wow! I'm really something. I never knew I was such a terrific person."

AFTERWORD

Now you've finished reading the book, and you know my thoughts and feelings on a lot of things, and specifically on energy. Now I'd like you to find out about your thoughts and feelings.

I want you to ask yourself a few questions:

1. Do you have physical energy?
   —Enough to play an hour of tennis and not feel you could drop dead?
   —Enough to clean your pad and be in a good, relaxed mood when your husband or wife or roomie comes home from work?
2. Are your nerves in good shape?

—Enough so you don't fly off the handle, get anxiety attacks, and yell at your spouse, kids, or pals?

—Enough so you don't get depressed and drag people around you?

3. Is your body in good shape?

—Enough so your posture is terrific and you walk tall?

—Enough so you really like to look at yourself in a full-length mirror?

4. Is your sex life happy?

—Enough that you smiled when you just thought about it?

—Enough that you harbor no guilt feelings *ever*?

5. Is your self-image a strong, positive one?

—Enough so you don't accept other people's negative opinions of you?

—Enough so you don't allow yourself to accept any creeping self-doubt?

6. Are you an overly critical person?

—Enough that you tend to passively criticize things instead of actively doing them?

—Enough that you regret certain things you've done in your life?

7. Are you a persistent person?

—Enough so that you've gotten most of the things in life you've really wanted?

—Enough that your determination will not let you take no for an answer for something you really want?

8. Are you a loving person?
   —Enough that you take really good care of yourself?
   —Enough that people care for you because they know you're a caring person?
9. Do you have a strong, healthy ego?
   —Enough that you rarely doubt yourself?
   —Enough that you believe you can accomplish anything you really set your mind and heart on?
10. Do you feel you really like yourself?
   —Enough that you hardly ever put yourself down?
   —Enough that of all the people you know, you can rely on yourself most of all?

1. How important is physical energy to you? After reading chapter 1, are you willing to try the yeast milkshake and vites for at least one month? Is having get-up-and-go what you want—the verve to do more, walk more, play more, have fun more? If after one month you don't feel absolutely superduper, what have you lost? Five minutes a day? It can't do you any harm, and remember my guarantee in chapter 1. It's absolute and unequivocal.

The very worst thing that can happen to you is you'll get healthy—or healthier—and have more energy than you ever dreamed possible.

So give it a try, and get ready to become a physical dynamo.

2. How important are calm nerves to you? Are you

willing to stop eating candy, sugared sodas, greasy donuts, cakes, pies, and cookies loaded with sugar, junk foods in general, and just plain sugar? Will you give up the martini syndrome? Can you kick the drug habit? (Ciggies and coffee are definitely drugs, no matter how much you'd like not to think so.) How extremely you will cut these things out of your life is an indication of how seriously good nerves and great health are to you. Sure, you can cut down and feel a little better—which is a step in the right direction; but if you want real results, cut 'em all out—and fast!

I once read, "You can have anything in life you want —it depends on what you're willing to give up for it."

3. How important is a physically attractive body—a good shape—to you? Are you willing to start a short (starting with one minute a day) exercise routine? Of course, if you've started the milkshake, you'll begin to have more energy and it'll be difficult *not* to walk more, play more and just *do* more. And the first-thing-in-the-morning breathing exercise will help your posture, will help you to stand tall. Think of what fun it'll be to put on a bikini and know the bod looks terrific. Just imagine standing in front of a mirror and really liking what you see—a body sans blubber and with an outline of form. It's not only good for your morale but for everyone associated with you. When people see what you've pulled off, it'll be an incentive for them to do it, too. It always takes somebody to start. So be the first on your block!

Aim high—nothing less than a gorgeous body. And

after all, it is possible. Just imagine what you'd look like if all the excess fat were trimmed away and your body lines were visible. Pretty neat, huh?

4. How important is a happy sex life to you? Are you willing to agree that between two consenting adults who care for each other anything goes, that guilt should be wiped out no matter what, because there's nothing to be guilty about? Once you can see sex objectively, as a body function like eating and drinking, you will see that only in excess or deficiency—as in all things—can any harm be done. Gorging yourself with food or starving your body are equally bad.

Objectively, sex is a body function necessary to physical health, and if physical health is one's aim in life, then sex should be understood and used. It is one of life's greatest sources of happiness, of which there sometimes seem to be too few; and so, as with all good things in life, learn to enjoy.

Take the person you care for and start to communicate. Find out what's the turn-on. You'll be amazed at how exciting it is to turn someone on, at how this becomes a turn-on for you. Ask questions. Show that you care. Have an open, two-way exchange of ideas. One of you has to start it—let it be you. The release of mental and emotional tension will be exhilarating, and once sex becomes free and loving between you, the physical release will be the happiest moment of your life.

5. How important is a strong, positive self-image to you? Are you willing to take a few minutes a day (you can

start with one) and do some mental exercises that will slowly change your belief in yourself from a negative to a positive one? Will you begin to train your mind to tune out every time a negative downer about yourself enters your mind? Just tune out the downer; no matter what it is, refuse to accept it. Keep your mind a vacuum and refuse to let any thought in. Hang on and just keep your mind a blank. Once you can do this and show your mind you're in control of it instead of vice versa, then you can make your mind think of something positive about yourself—what you want to be or what you want to do. The whole point is that your self-image is just that—a *self*-image, dictated to your mind by *you*. So once you're in control of your mind, you can dictate to your mind exactly what you want. Are you willing to do it?

6. How important is it to you not to be overly critical? Are you willing to stop criticizing everything in your life, including yourself? If there's something you don't like, either change it or learn to live with it, but don't be a vocal critic. And when the urge comes to look back and regret something you've done, will you be able to say to yourself that you did it for a specific reason at the time and nothing you can do now can change it? So even though you maybe wouldn't do the same thing again, you recognize it can't be changed and you're where you are today because you did it. If you'd done something else your whole life would be different—and maybe lots worse! Every action is a link in the chain of life, and if one is changed it can change the whole course of life.

7. How important is being persistent to you? Are you willing to give up procrastinating, waiting till tomorrow to do it? The thing that's missing if you're not a determined person is the clear-cut desire for something. We usually have a fuzzy idea of what we more or less want out of life, but those who are determined know exactly what they want and where they want to go. I mean, how can you be determined if something's fuzzy?

So to become persistent, you must know precisely what it is you want. And there are ways of finding out. How about taking that aptitude test I talked about earlier? Call your city library and ask where they give them. And after you take one, sit by yourself and really try to figure out what would make you happiest to be doing the rest of your life. Once you make your decision, you're on your way. You won't believe how persistent you'll be once you know what you really want.

"MAN, KNOW THYSELF." Aristotle was the wisest of men. Just become a little introspective for a short while and become acquainted with your self. Because your self, the deepest part of you, your subconscious (or Giant Self, as I call it), knows where you should be if you'll just listen. And when you're listening, you'll get your chance to be persistent. Keep listening till you come up with the answers—and you will, if you just don't give up.

8. How important is being loving to you? Are you willing to start really taking good care of yourself first and then to start caring about life around you? Can you train yourself to realize that until *you* are cared for by

you, it's impossible to truly care for something or somebody else? Look at the mother who sacrifices her life for her children and then is crushed when they grow up and resent her. She lived only for them. She never cared what she looked like as long as the kids were well dressed, so she looked ratty and embarrassed them. She never cared what she did as long as they had a good time, so she was a bore. She ate junk herself but made sure the kids took their vites and drank their milk. She felt awful a lot of the time and couldn't help nagging—didn't they know it was for their own good? No wonder they resent her. She unconsciously considers them her possessions. Didn't she give everything up for them?

It just doesn't work.

"To THINE OWN SELF BE TRUE." You must care for yourself first; and then you can't help caring for others, because you'll be happy. If you believe God or Spirit or Love or Something created you, and She/He/It is intelligent and cared enough for you to create you, then isn't it sort of a duty you owe She/He/It to care for you too?

But you can't give what isn't there. So to put love in your life, first learn to care for yourself, and automatically there will be enough love in your heart to spread around to everyone and everything that enters your world.

And how to love yourself? First make sure your body is healthy, and work at it. Work at it as much as you work at your job, because it's far more important than your job. It's your life. Think of yourself. Don't be afraid of being introspective. Turn your eyes inward and ask yourself questions about yourself. Believe me, your subconscious or Giant Self or Spirit knows what you need if you'll only listen. You give so much time to others and other things. Give a little time to yourself. Even if you start with one minute a day when you first wake up, or on your coffee break—or Sanka break, if you really care!—and build up gradually!

Naturally, no extreme is good. Narcissism is bad enough, but the other extreme is even worse. Try to do good things for yourself. Substitute yogurt for ice cream, knowing you're building health. Substitute busyness for smoking and Sanka for coffee and know that you're thinking of yourself first for a change. It'll feel so good that the people around you will notice you're in a better mood and you're even nicer. Selfmoreness instead of selflessness. Believe me, your self is all you got, and if you don't treat it well, no one else will either.

People take you at your own evaluation, and if you evaluate yourself to be a worthwhile person, everyone you meet will, too. They'll treat you better, you'll treat them better, and love will ripple and spread.

9. How important is it to you to have a strong, healthy ego? Are you willing to make an effort to try and accomplish something in your life that will build up your self-esteem? Because that's the common denominator in all strong, healthy egos. No one is born with it. Sure, we're all the center of our own little universes when we're infants, and mommy runs when we yell, and we're pretty much little dictators. But we learn soon enough as we

grow older that mommy and poppy ain't gonna drop everything when we want it—and it's a rude awakening. So our little egos get deflated as soon as we are not completely dependent on adults.

Everyone's self-esteem is built on accomplishment, be it baking a fantastic cake, growing a gorgeous rose tree, writing a superb screenplay, becoming the best bossa-nova-er in the neighborhood, playing a wild trumpet, driving the most expensive car, or having the biggest bankroll. Of course, the ego predicated on money alone is tenuous and shaky. What happens if you blow the money and can't re-earn it? But talent nurtured and developed is a lasting ego trip, and one in which you truly believe you deserve the praise because it's something you have worked at and accomplished.

Everyone I interviewed (and they're all accomplishers) —everyone, without exception, said they had a strong, healthy ego. When I asked to what this was attributed, everyone, without exception, said because of his or her accomplishment. David Susskind, Buddy Rich, Arlene Dahl, Alex Cohen, Virginia Graham, Sheila MacRae, Jim Bouton, Dr. Joyce Brothers, Percy Sutton, Sammy Cahn, Walter Blum, Hildegarde, Henny Youngman, Monique Van Vooren, Dr. Benjamin Frank, Serge Obolensky, and many others—everyone said that until some accomplishment was attained, the ego was not strong.

However, most said they knew they had to do something; it was a driving force. In fact, you might say their egos were on the weak side and that fear of being a nothing was the driving force to become something—to do something important. Well, not everyone has to be a star. We don't all have the same needs and desires. For some of us, stardom is the only answer and for others of us, knitting a beautiful afghan or working with a retarded child and having success in communicating and teaching him or her to be self-reliant is enough to make us feel important.

But know one thing. You must *do* something. Not talk about it or think about it, but do it. And if you follow through on this, be assured that the better you do it, the stronger and healthier your ego will become, and the happier you will be.

10. How important is it to you to really like yourself? Are you willing to accept the idea that liking oneself is the basis of all happiness? Just stop and analyze what I'm saying. It's a pretty positive statement, no? But I know it to be true. If you do like yourself, that means you're doing things and they're worthwhile things. We can't lie to ourselves or kid ourselves about being happy. We know we are or we aren't, right? We can lie to ourselves or kid ourselves about a lot of things, but not about being happy. Either we are or we're not. Now if we're happy we're doing things that we feel are worthwhile; and if we're doing things we feel are worthwhile, then we must be worthwhile for doing them. And if we're worthwhile, we like ourselves.

Again, pick out a few worthwhile, easy things you can do to benefit yourself. Like cutting down on the cups of coffee drunk in a day, or the martinis, or cigarettes. Even if you cut out only a quarter of the amount, it's something, and it will make you like yourself a little better for the willpower exerted. And God knows you will be better off with two cups of coffee less, or five cigarettes less, or two martinis less. Or walk two extra blocks down to another bus stop instead of the usual closer one. You know you can use the exercise, and maybe in a week or so you'll walk four blocks, then six, until you're really getting a lot of painless exercise and feeling lots better, physically and mentally. Or promise yourself that the next time your husband starts picking on you, you'll just look up at him and smile and say nothing. That's a rough one, but not impossible, and what a good feeling of self-control it'll give you. Or organize a bunch of guys in the neighborhood to form a barbershop quartet. Singing is fun and good exercise; you have to have breath control to sing.

There are so many little worthwhile things you can do if you just stop and figure them out. We're all individuals and have different needs to be satisfied. But if you start to satisfy yourself by doing things for yourself, you'll find you're much less dependent on others for your happiness, and that's a good place to be. Self-reliance is a peaceful state. No matter what anyone does or says, you know you'll get along. And you'll like yourself for being independent.

———◆———

I've been helped by many people and many books, and if I, in turn, through this book, have helped you maybe a little and hopefully a lot, I'd like to hear from you about how you've changed your life.

Write to me c/o

Hawthorn Books
260 Madison Avenue
New York, New York 10016

The one thing more than anything else I wish for every one of you is that you will *expect* to have everything in life you want . . . you won't let guilt or fear get in your way, and that you will know—not believe or think or feel—but *know* that you deserve everything in life you want. And when you realize that your SOURCE is good, or God, or your Giant Self, or whatever name you give the goodness within you, you will *have* everything in life you want.